Periocular Rejuvenation

Guest Editor

EDWARD H. FARRIOR, MD

FACIAL PLASTIC SURGERY CLINICS OF NORTH AMERICA

www.facialplastic.theclinics.com

August 2010 • Volume 18 • Number 3

SAUNDERS an imprint of ELSEVIER, Inc.

W.B. SAUNDERS COMPANY
A Division of Elsevier Inc.

1600 John F. Kennedy Blvd., Suite 1800, Philadelphia, PA 19103-2899

http://www.theclinics.com

FACIAL PLASTIC SURGERY CLINICS OF NORTH AMERICA Volume 18, Number 3
August 2010 ISSN 1064-7406, ISBN 978-1-4377-2448-6

Editor: Joanne Husovski

Facial Plastic Surgery Clinics of North America (ISSN 1064-7406) is published quarterly by Elsevier Inc., 360 Park Avenue South, New York, NY 10010-1710. Months of issue are February, May, August, and November. Business and Editorial Offices: 1600 John F. Kennedy Blvd., Suite 1800, Philadelphia, PA 19103-2899. Periodicals postage paid at New York, NY, and additional mailing offices. Subscription prices are $306.00 per year (US individuals), $437.00 per year (US institutions), $344.00 per year (Canadian individuals), $524.00 per year (Canadian institutions), $412.00 per year (foreign individuals), $524.00 per year (foreign institutions), $149.00 per year (US students), and $207.00 per year (foreign students). Foreign air speed delivery is included in all *Clinics* subscription prices. All prices are subject to change without notice. POSTMASTER: Send address changes to *Facial Plastic Surgery Clinics*, Elsevier Health Sciences Division, Subscription Customer Service, 3251 Riverport Lane, Maryland Heights, MO 63043. **Customer service: 1-800-654-2452 (US and Canada); 1-314-447-8871 (outside US and Canada); Fax: 314-447-8029; E-mail:journalscustomerservice-usa@elsevier.com (for print support); journalsonline support-usa@elsevier.com (for online support).**

Reprints. For copies of 100 or more of articles in this publication, please contact the Commercial Reprints Department, Elsevier Inc., 360 Park Avenue South, New York, NY 10010-1710. Tel.: 212-633-3812; Fax: 212-462-1935; E-mail: reprints@elsevier.com.

Facial Plastic Surgery Clinics of North America is covered in *MEDLINE/PubMed* (*Index Medicus*).

Printed and bound by CPI Group (UK) Ltd, Croydon, CR0 4YY

Transferred to Digital Print 2011

Contributors

CONSULTING EDITOR

J. REGAN THOMAS, MD, FACS
Professor and Chairman, Department of
Otolaryngology, University of Illinois at
Chicago, Chicago, Illinois

EDITORIAL BOARD

SHAN R. BAKER, MD
Professor and Chief, Section of Plastic and
Reconstructive Surgery, University of
Michigan, Ann Arbor, Michigan

ROBERT KELLMAN, MD
Professor and Chairman, Department of
Otolaryngology, State University of New York
Upstate Medical University, Syracuse,
New York

RUSSELL W.H. KRIDEL, MD
Clinical Associate Professor, Department
of Otolaryngology–Head and Neck Surgery,
Division of Facial Plastic Surgery, University
of Texas Health Science Center, Houston,
Texas

STEPHEN W. PERKINS, MD
Private Practitioner, Perkins Facial Plastic
Surgery, Indianapolis, Indiana

ANTHONY P. SCLAFANI, MD, FACS
Director of Facial Plastic Surgery,
The New York Eye and Ear Infirmary,
New York, New York; and Professor of
Otolaryngology–Head and Neck Surgery,
New York Medical College, Valhalla,
New York

GUEST EDITOR

EDWARD H. FARRIOR, MD
Visiting Associate Clinical Professor,
Department of Otolaryngology, The University
of Virginia, Charlottesville, Virginia; Associate
Clinical Professor, Department of
Otolaryngology, University of South Florida,
Tampa, Florida

AUTHORS

BRADFORD BADER, MD
Fellow, Division of Facial Plastic and
Reconstructive Surgery, Department of
Otolaryngology–Head and Neck Surgery,
The Ohio State University Medical Center,
Columbus, Ohio

EDWARD D. BUCKINGHAM, MD
Buckingham Center for Facial Plastic Surgery,
Austin, Texas

EDWARD H. FARRIOR, MD
Visiting Associate Clinical Professor,
Department of Otolaryngology, The University
of Virginia, Charlottesville, Virginia; Associate
Clinical Professor, Department of
Otolaryngology, University of South Florida,
Tampa, Florida

JONATHAN R. GRANT, MD
Dedham, Massachusetts

LAURA HETZLER, MD
Division of Facial Plastic and Reconstructive
Surgery, Department of Otolaryngology–Head
and Neck Surgery, University of California,
Davis, Sacramento, California

AMIR M. KARAM, MD
Director, Carmel Valley Facial Plastic
Surgery; Clinical Faculty, Division of
Otolaryngology–Head and Neck, Department
of Surgery; University of California, San Diego
School of Medicine, San Diego, California

KEITH A. LAFERRIERE, MD, FACS
Facial Plastic Surgery, St John's Clinic,
Springfield, Missouri

SAMUEL M. LAM, MD, FACS
Director, Willow Bend Wellness Center,
Lam Facial Plastic Surgery Center and Hair
Restoration Institute, Plano, Texas

LILY P. LOVE, MD
Facial Plastic and Reconstructive Surgeon,
Otolaryngology, Facial Plastic and
Reconstructive Surgery, Cedars Sinai Medical
Group, Los Angeles, California

WILLIAM P. MACK, MD
Clinical Assistant Professor of Opthamology,
Division of Oculoplastics, University of South
Florida, Tampa, Florida

SAM P. MOST, MD
Division of Facial Plastic and Reconstructive
Surgery, Department of Otolaryngology–Head
and Neck Surgery, Stanford University
School of Medicine, Stanford, California

SACHIN PARIKH, MD
Division of Facial Plastic and Reconstructive
Surgery, Department of Otolaryngology–Head
and Neck Surgery, Stanford University
School of Medicine, Stanford, California

STEPHEN P. SMITH, MD
Director, Division of Facial Plastic and
Reconstructive Surgery, Assistant Professor,
Department of Otolaryngology–Head and
Neck Surgery, The Ohio State University
Medical Center, Columbus, Ohio

JONATHAN SYKES, MD
Director of Facial Plastic and Reconstructive
Surgery, Department of Otolaryngology–Head
and Neck Surgery, University of California,
Davis, Sacramento, California

EDWIN F. WILLIAMS III, MD, FACS
Facial Plastic and Reconstructive Surgery,
Williams Center Plastic Surgery Specialists,
Latham; Clinical Professor of Surgery,
Facial Plastic and Reconstructive
Surgery, Division of Otolaryngology–Head
and Neck Surgery, Department of
Surgery, Albany Medical Center,
Albany, New York

CORY C. YEH, MD
Facial Plastic and Reconstructive Surgery,
Yeh Facial Plastic Surgery, Laguna Woods,
California

Contents

Midface Restoration in the Management of the Lower Eyelid   365

Cory C. Yeh and Edwin F. Williams III

> Aging of the midface and lower eyelid represents one of the earliest clinically detect-able areas of aging on the face. These senile changes include laxity of eyelid skin, pseudoherniation of orbital fat, ptosis of the suborbicularis oculi and malar fat pads, and loss of facial volume. Several approaches, including surgical and nonsur-gical procedures, have been developed to counter the effects of aging on the mid-face and lower eyelid. This article reviews the techniques used by the authors to rejuvenate the midface and lower eyelid, and illustrates a comprehensive approach to management of this complex facial region.

The Brow and Forehead in Periocular Rejuvenation   375

Laura Hetzler and Jonathan Sykes

> Recognition of the brow as an integral contributor to periocular appearance im-proves and prolongs results from facial rejuvenation surgery. The approach to the brow and forehead in periocular rejuvenation must be chosen on an individual basis. The approaches discussed require in-depth knowledge of complex forehead and temporal anatomy to navigate the planes and important neurovascular structures safely. This article discusses anatomy, preoperative evaluation and considerations, surgical techniques, and complications in rejuvenation of forehead and brow.

Autologous Fat and Fillers in Periocular Rejuvenation   385

Edward D. Buckingham, Bradford Bader, and Stephen P. Smith

> Facial volume loss is an important component of facial aging, especially in the peri-ocular region. The authors evaluate the normal and aging anatomy of the periocular region and then discuss volume restoration of this region using hyaluronic acid, cal-cium hydroxylapatite, and autologous fat transfer. Preoperative assessment, oper-ative technique, postoperative care, and complications are addressed.

Periocular Rejuvenation: Lower Eyelid Blepharoplasty with Fat Repositioning and the Suborbicularis Oculi Fat   399

Jonathan R. Grant and Keith A. LaFerriere

> Treatment of the aging lower eyelid is determined by the anatomic variables noted for each surgical candidate. Although surgeons have traditionally consid-ered dermatochalasis, fat pseudoherniation, and eyelid position as the main treat-ment objectives in lower blepharoplasty, the vector of the infraorbital rim and the anterior plane of the cornea, tear trough, and aging in the midface also merit critical consideration. In this article, indications and technical aspects, the trans-conjunctival and external approaches, fat excision versus fat repositioning, and suborbicularis oculi fat lifting and fat transplantation are discussed and the authors' preference for the various methods of lower blepharoplasty is presented. Common adjunct procedures used to supplement lower blepharoplasty tech-niques and the role of injectable fillers in periocular rejuvenation are also mentioned.

Facial Plastic Surgery Clinics of North America

THE CLINICS ARE NOW AVAILABLE ONLINE!

Access your subscription at:
www.theclinics.com

Preface

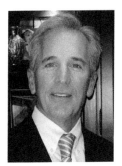

Edward H. Farrior, MD
Guest Editor

The revolution and evolution in periorbital rejuvenation has had no rival in facial plastic and reconstructive surgery in the past decade. Volumization and fat preservation have led the changes in our approach to the periorbita. It is now almost universally accepted that the full lid and periorbita represent a more youthful and healthy appearance. The evolution in the management of the lower lid started with the mobilization and suspension of the suborbicularis osculi fat (SOOF) and the repositioning of the orbital fat and has progressed to the use of autologous fat and synthetic fillers to address the nasal-jugal groove and shallow periorbita.

In this issue of *Facial Plastic Surgery Clinics* we have assembled an esteemed group of authors to help make sense of the evolution in management of the periorbita and help the reader develop his or her own decision-making pathway for addressing the aging process. This process must first and foremost consider the normal anatomy and function of the eyelid. Their preservation during any and all interventions must be paramount. Being able to identify abnormalities of form and function preoperatively will help the surgeon avoid complications. Surgical and nonsurgical options in rejuvenation will be provided for the reader's consideration. The goal is to provide readers with a reference that covers the treatment options available for the rejuvenation of this complex and vital anatomic region of the face and help them to better serve their patients.

Edward H. Farrior, MD
Department of Otolaryngology
The University of Virginia
Charlottesville, VA, USA

Department of Otolaryngology
University of South Florida
2908 Azeele Street
Tampa, FL 33609, USA

E-mail address:
efarrior@tampabay.rr.com

Facial Plast Surg Clin N Am 18 (2010) ix
doi:10.1016/j.fsc.2010.05.003
1064-7406/10/$ – see front matter © 2010 Elsevier Inc. All rights reserved.

facialplastic.theclinics.com

Midface Restoration in the Management of the Lower Eyelid

Cory C. Yeh, MD[a],*, Edwin F. Williams III, MD[b,c]

KEYWORDS

- Midface • Lower eyelid • Lipotransfer
- Fat transfer • Facial rejuvenation

Rejuvenation of the aging face has undergone significant transformation over the past 20 years. Collective understanding of the physiologic forces of aging on skin, soft tissue, and facial bony structures has permitted the development of various surgical and nonsurgical treatments to correct or limit these effects. Further, increased understanding of the importance of volume restoration in facial rejuvenation has improved the results of interventions and addressed a critical component of aging that was previously ignored. Although almost all aspects of facial plastic surgery have significantly evolved during this time, restoration of the aging midface has been particularly rewarding for most surgeons and patients. This article seeks to describe the importance of midface restoration, the evolution of various treatments that have been developed, a synopsis of the authors' current approach to rejuvenation of the midface complex, and the role of midface restoration in the management of the aging lower lid.

The anatomy of the midface has been well described by many investigators but often lacks clearly described anatomic boundaries. To simplify discussion on this topic, the midface is defined as an inverted triangular volume of tissue bordered laterally by a line drawn from the lateral canthus to the oral commissure and medially by a line drawn through the nasolabial fold from the medial canthus. Anatomically, this complex contains the lower sling of the orbicularis oculi muscle, orbicularis and zygomaticocutaneous retaining ligaments, the suborbicularis oculi fat (SOOF) pad, and the malar fat pad. One of the most challenging aspects encountered in the study of the midface is a thorough understanding of the relationship of the midface to the lower lid. It is difficult to know precisely where the lower lid ends and where the midface begins.[1] Even so, the authors have found that a precise anatomic separation between these 2 structures is often unnecessary, because it is the combined rejuvenation of the midface and lower lid complex that results in optimal aesthetic rejuvenation. For the authors, this concept of zonal rejuvenation has become a key driving force to obtaining natural results, and has resulted in improved midface restoration.

Aging of the midface and lower lid complex is a continual process that involves changes to the skin, soft tissue, and bony facial structures. Many women and men show clinical signs of aging to the midface and lower lid in their late 30s, making this one of the earliest detectable areas of facial aging and, consequently, one of the initial areas of patient concern. Aging of the midface and lower eyelid skin is largely exacerbated by environmental effects that include solar damage, as well as the formation of rhytids caused by

[a] Facial Plastic and Reconstructive Surgery, Yeh Facial Plastic Surgery, 24331 El Toro Road, Suite 350, Laguna Woods, CA 92637, USA
[b] Facial Plastic and Reconstructive Surgery, Williams Center Plastic Surgery Specialists, 1072 Troy-Schenectady Road, Latham, NY 12110, USA
[c] Facial Plastic and Reconstructive Surgery, Division of Otolaryngology–Head and Neck Surgery, Department of Surgery, Albany Medical Center, Albany, NY 12208, USA
* Corresponding author.
E-mail address: coryyeh@gmail.com

Facial Plast Surg Clin N Am 18 (2010) 365–374
doi:10.1016/j.fsc.2010.04.001
1064-7406/10/$ – see front matter © 2010 Elsevier Inc. All rights reserved.

repeated muscular contractions. Soft-tissue changes to the midface and lower lid include a weakening of the orbital retaining ligaments and an inferior displacement of the zygomaticocutaneous ligament (**Fig. 1**). These changes are thought to be largely caused by the gravitational effect on facial soft tissue.[2] A direct result of this effect is vertical displacement of the lower eyelid and the loss of a youthful-appearing, short, and full eyelid.[3] A youthful eyelid should be free of tarsal ligament laxity, with strong tone and an adequate septum that resists pseudoherniation of the orbital fat, whereas a youthful midface should demonstrate adequate vertical height of the SOOF and malar fat pads, providing support to the malar area.

One of the most important and previously overlooked features of an aged midface and lower lid is the loss of facial volume. This process is thought to be secondary to atrophy of the SOOF and malar fat pads. As a result of these changes, the midface and lower lid appears deflated, flat, and hollow, exacerbating the underlying bony facial structure. The periorbital changes described above are observed in continuity with deepening of the nasolabial fold and ptosis of the midface with vertical descent of the SOOF and malar fat pad.[4,5] The combined result of these aging changes creates a loss of facial width in the malar region, a tear trough deformity, and the projection of a tired appearance (**Fig. 2**).

One of the earliest interventions in countering the effects of midface aging was a surgical approach to specifically address the ptotic fat pads and soft tissue. A historical review of surgical midface lifts has recently been published.[2] The senior author (E.F.W.) employed an endoscopic subperiosteal approach to the midface in the mid

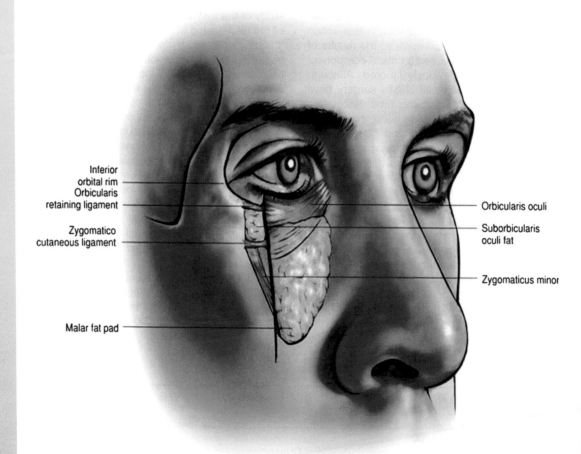

Fig. 1. Aging of the midface and lower lid results in weakening of the orbicularis oculi muscle sling and the gravitational descent of the SOOF and malar fat pads. *Reprinted from* Krishna S, Williams EF 3rd. Lipocontouring in conjunction with the minimal incision brow and subperiosteal midface lift: the next dimension in midface rejuvenation. Facial Plast Surg Clin North Am 2006;14(3):222; with permission.

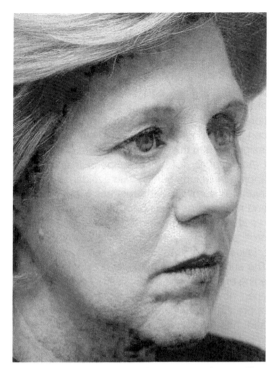

Fig. 2. Clinical features of aging in the midface include a loss of malar width, a tear trough deformity, skeletonized orbital rim, and prominent nasolabial fold. (*From* Pontius AT, Williams EF 3rd. The extended minimal incision approach to midface rejuvenation. Facial Plast Surg Clin North Am 2005;13(3):411–9; with permission.)

1990s after careful consideration of the physiologic effects of aging as well as of the safety of the technique. As described by Ramirez,[6] the endoscopic midface lift involves careful elevation of the SOOF pad with the underlying periosteum along the inferior orbital rim and malar areas by creating a dissection plane between the malar-zygomatic arch and the temporal pocket. The experience gained from endoscopic brow lifting and from the management of bony facial trauma in a subperiosteal plane has made this approach familiar to many facial plastic surgeons. Additional considerations such as the importance of maintaining a safe lower lid and attaining adequate visualization of the midface were paramount in the development of this particular technique.

SUBPERIOSTEAL MIDFACE LIFT

A complete description of subperiosteal midface lift has already been published,[7] and a summary is given here. The patient is administered anesthesia either via intravenous sedation or general anesthesia. Appropriate preparation consists of securing the patient's hair tufts with brown paper

tape and the marking of standard endoscopic incisions. If a brow lift is to be performed at the same time, endoscopic brow lift incisions are marked with a 2-cm incision in the midline, 2 2-cm incisions located lateral to the midline in a paramedian position (approximately at the lateral canthus) just posterior to the hairline, and 2 additional 3- to 4-cm incisions located over the temporal region and extending over a 4-cm distance above the helical crus and over the temporalis muscle and fascia (**Fig. 3**). After infiltration of local anesthetic (1% lidocaine with 1:100,000 epinephrine) to the incision sites and midface, surgical incision is performed along the marked incisions, and an endoscopic brow lift, if planned, is performed by subperiosteal release of the brow through the midline and paramedian incisions with suture resuspension through cortical bone tunnels. For the midface, the planned temporal incision is made down to the level of the temporoparietal fascia (TPF), and dissection is performed with a blunt elevator over the true temporalis fascia. Dissection is performed downward to the orbital rim and the arcus marginalis is released from the superolateral orbital rim near the lateral canthus with the periosteal elevator. Further dissection is then made inferiorly toward the midface by entering the temporal fat pad and releasing the periosteal attachments over the zygomatic arch itself, with careful attention paid to avoid injury to the overlying frontal branch of the facial nerve. The subperiosteal dissection is then continued inferiorly over the malar eminence to release the zygomaticus major and minor muscular attachments and malar fat pad from the underlying malar bone (**Fig. 4**). This dissection is performed until the midfacial structures are adequately released, but unintended masseteric elevation is unnecessary because it can lead to trismus and spasm. Suture suspension of the midface soft

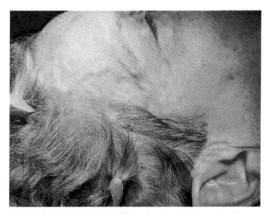

Fig. 3. Access to the midface in an endoscopic subperiosteal approach is through a 4-cm–long temporoparietal incision just posterior to the hairline.

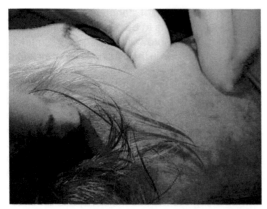

Fig. 4. Elevation of the midfacial soft tissue is accomplished with a blunt elevator in the subperiosteal plane.

tissue is then performed to the temporalis fascia with a vertically oriented vector to minimize distortion of the lateral canthus (**Fig. 5**). Redundant temporalis soft tissue is pulled superolaterally by suturing the TPF just anterior to the temporoparietal incision to the temporalis fascia, and closure is performed with surgical staples.

A review of the authors' experience with subperiosteal midface lifting was performed, which involved a retrospective review of 325 charts for complications as well as determination of a facial aesthetic rating for various facial zones postoperatively.[8] In this study, zone I included the malar complex, zone II included the nasolabial sulcus, and zone III included the jaw line. Results from this study indicated significant improvement in zone I (70% marked, 30% mild) and zone III

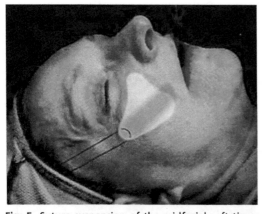

Fig. 5. Suture suspension of the midfacial soft tissue to the temporalis fascia. *Reprinted from* Pontius AT, Williams EF 3rd. The extended minimal incision approach to midface rejuvenation. Facial Plast Surg Clin North Am 2005;13(3):416; with permission.

(30% marked, 50% mild), with less than optimal results for zone II (60% mild, 36% no improvement). The study also confirmed the rarity of complications following subperiosteal midface lift, which included subperiosteal abscess, neuropraxia of the facial nerve, and prolonged edema of the midface. In addition, lateral canthal distortion after subperiosteal midface lift, a valid concern among many surgeons, was found to be insignificant in this study population.

Advantages of the subperiosteal midface approach include safety, with avoidance of direct injury to neurovascular structures over the temple and midface. As described, the approach can be readily adapted to address the midface, temporal area, and brow simultaneously, thereby achieving rejuvenation of the upper two-thirds of the face. The subperiosteal midface lift results in the tightening of the orbicularis sling with a resultant shortened lower eyelid (**Fig. 6**). In addition, this approach directly repositions the malar fat pad and has also been shown to result in some improvement of the ptotic tissue of the upper jowl (**Fig. 7**). Limitations of this procedure include the possibility of temporary lateral canthal overtightening, but unlike the direct transconjunctival approach, a lateral canthopexy is not required and permanent lateral canthal distortion with rounding or various degrees of ectropion can be avoided.[9] Other limitations include dimpling of the skin at the sites of suture suspension if placed too superficially, limited results in patients with poor bony structure and thick, round faces, and the possibility of subtle postoperative results.

In the early 2000s, the senior author (E.F.W.) performed a critical evaluation of the endoscopic subperiosteal approach to the midface. Despite the safety of the procedure and wide patient acceptance, it was clear that this technique alone was incompletely addressing the aging midface. The inadequacies of this procedure and others were particularly evident in the interface between the lower eyelids and midface. Research and careful analysis by many investigators helped to illustrate that a key component of aging that was not being appropriately improved through this subperiosteal transtemporal lift was volume restoration. The concept of gradual volume loss of facial soft tissue, as well as facial bony resorption of the midface, was a critical step in formulating a comprehensive approach to the midface. In recognition of the importance of this physiologic change in the aging midface, the authors' group turned to facial lipotransfer to restore volumetric loss. As initially described by Coleman,[10] autologous facial lipotransfer provides a reliable soft-tissue augmentation to volume-deficient areas of the face.

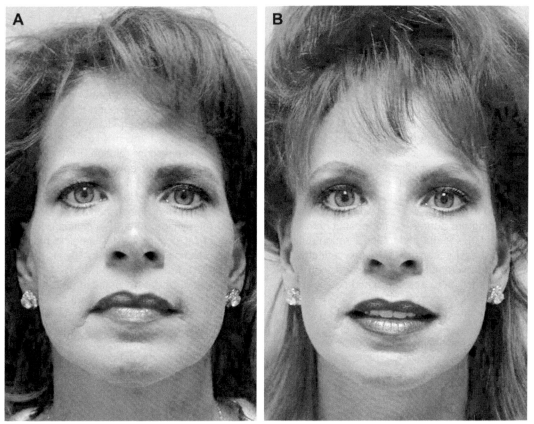

Fig. 6. (*A*) Preoperative photograph of a woman, demonstrating a ptotic midface. (*B*) Postoperative photograph 1 year after subperiosteal midface lift, demonstrating improvement along the malar eminence.

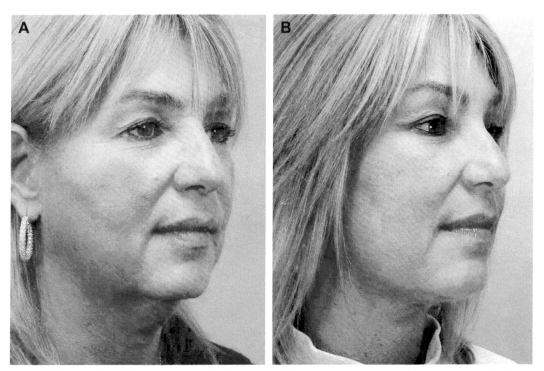

Fig. 7. (*A*) Preoperative oblique photograph of a woman, demonstrating an aged midface secondary to descent of the SOOF and malar fat pads. (*B*) Postoperative oblique photograph 1 year after subperiosteal midface lift, demonstrating restoration of midfacial soft tissue after suture suspension.

Autologous facial lipotransfer is a technique that involves the meticulous placement of the patient's own fat into areas of the face that demonstrate clinical volume loss. In the authors' experience, the most significant improvement in postoperative results occurs when addressing the midface and lower lid complex together. Addressing them together is important because the volume loss of the midface and lower lid does not occur in isolation from each other but represents a continuum of volumetric change across the periocular region. Once the other existing components of lower eyelid aging are addressed (ie, pseudoherniation of ocular fat), volume restoration through autologous lipotransfer can be extremely effective in promoting a youthful-appearing, short, and fuller eyelid, in addition to a restored midface.

AUTOLOGOUS FACIAL LIPOTRANSFER

A complete description of autologous facial lipotransfer has been published,[11] and a summary is given here. The patient is administered anesthesia either via intravenous sedation or general anesthesia. Areas of facial volume loss in the lower lid and midface complex are carefully marked before surgical manipulation. Although the procedure is tailored to the individual patient, in general most patients receive a total of 5 to 20 mL of fat in each side. A tumescent solution (1 mL of 1% lidocaine with 1:100,000 epinephrine, 4 mL of 1% plain lidocaine, and 15 mL of isotonic sodium chloride) is injected to the donor site (ie, abdomen or thigh) through a long liposuction cannula attached to a 20-mL syringe. After 15 minutes, donor harvesting of fat occurs with a tunneling maneuver and the solution is collected in 10-mL Luer-Lok syringes (BD, Franklin Lakes, NJ, USA). After the centrifugation of fat to remove the nonviable adipocytes, blood, and tumescent solution, the fat is placed into the marked areas with 1-mL syringes attached to a 16-gauge blunt cannula. The fat is injected slowly, in multiple passes, particularly along the infraorbital rim, to avoid

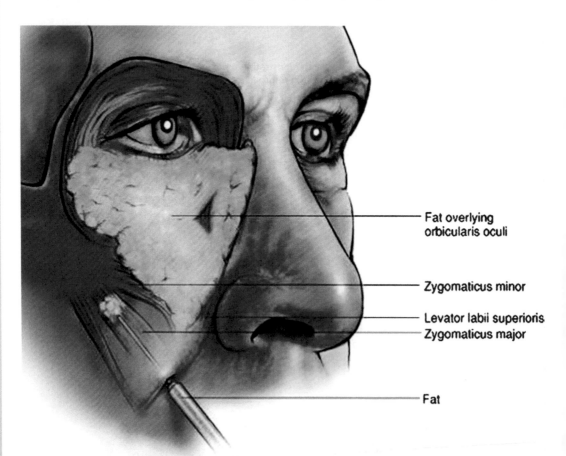

Fat overlying orbicularis oculi

Zygomaticus minor

Levator labii superioris
Zygomaticus major

Fat

Fig. 8. Autologous lipotransfer procedure with placement of fat to the lower lid and midface complex through a blunt cannula. *Reprinted from* DeFatta RJ, Williams EF 3rd. Fat transfer in conjunction with facial rejuvenation procedures. Facial Plast Surg Clin North Am 2008;16(4):386; with permission.

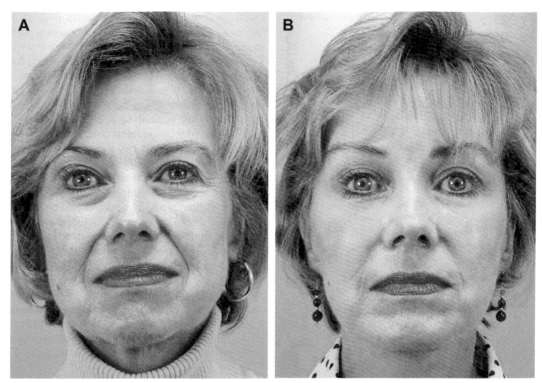

Fig. 9. (A) Preoperative photograph of a woman, demonstrating skeletonization of the orbital rim with significant loss of periorbital volume. (B) Postoperative photograph 1 year after lipotransfer, demonstrating improvement as a result of volume restoration.

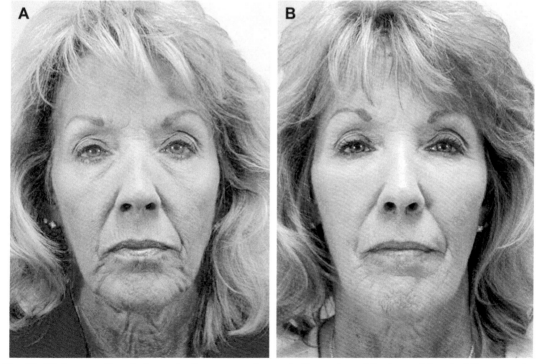

Fig. 10. (A) Preoperative photograph of a woman, demonstrating aging of the lower lid and midface complex. (B) Postoperative photograph 1 year after lipotransfer, demonstrating improvement with volume correction of the inferior orbital rim, nasojugal fold, and malar eminence.

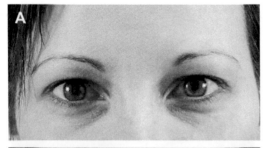

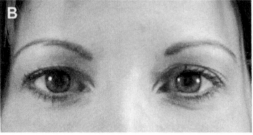

Fig. 11. (*A*) Preprocedure photograph of a woman, demonstrating a tear trough deformity. (*B*) Postprocedure photograph after injection of 1 vial of Restylane, demonstrating correction of the tear trough deformity.

postoperative palpable abnormalities (**Fig. 8**). In addition, depth of placement is critical in a plane deep to the orbicularis muscle.

Advantages of fat transfer are numerous, and include a sufficient supply of adipose tissue in most patients. It is a less expensive procedure than other dermal fillers, because the material is provided by the patient, fat is biocompatible and safe, tissue reaction is minimal, donor harvesting is straightforward, and there appear to be long-lasting effects of volume restoration (**Fig. 9**). Potential limitations include infection, asymmetry of fat placement, palpable abnormalities, granuloma formation, prolonged edema, and unpredictable resorption. The authors have found that many of these limitations seem to be technique-dependent and can be minimized through careful attention to placement in the appropriate tissue plane.

To critically review the results in their practice, the authors' group conducted a study that compared the aesthetic results of a midface lift with simultaneous fat transfer to a midface lift alone.[12] Multiple facial zones were analyzed including the tear trough and infraorbital rim, the malar eminence, the

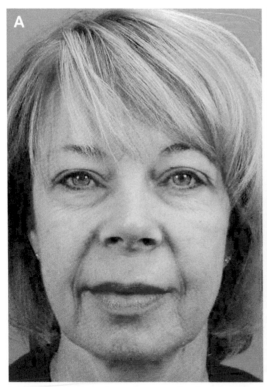

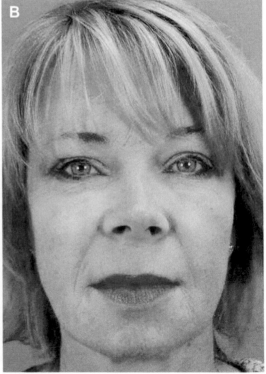

Fig. 12. (*A*) Preprocedure photograph of a woman, demonstrating skeletonization of the inferior orbital rim, deep nasojugal fold, and flattened midface. (*B*) Postprocedure photograph after injection of 4 vials of Radiesse, demonstrating improvement to the lower lid and midface complex.

submalar region, and the nasolabial crease. Results indicated that the tear trough, infraorbital rim, and the nasolabial crease were significantly improved when volume in the form of autologous fat was added to these areas. At present, the authors perform autologous lipotransfer concomitantly with a subperiosteal midface lift to specific areas of the lower lid and midface that demonstrate volume loss (**Fig. 10**). These areas are, for the most part, consistent and include the tear trough, infraorbital rim, malar eminence, and nasolabial crease.[13]

Volume restoration can also be achieved through the injection of various dermal fillers. Restylane (Medicis Pharmaceutical Corporation, Scottsdale, AZ, USA), a hyaluronic acid dermal filler, is a viable alternative to autologous fat for the purpose of restoring facial volume in the periocular region. The authors' group has found that Restylane is forgiving when placed in the appropriate dermal depth deep to the orbicularis muscle sling. The authors prefer to use Restylane in the tear trough particularly when there is a severe type V deformity present, but frequently avoid its use in the midface soft tissue because the volume required is often

more than a 1 or 2 vials (**Fig. 11**). For midface volume loss, the authors often use Radiesse (Bioform Medical Inc, San Mateo, CA, USA), a calcium hydroxyapatite dermal filler, to restore soft-tissue volume loss. The authors are careful to avoid close placement to the orbital rim but believe Radiesse provides a better foundation for volume over the medial and lateral boundaries of the midface (**Fig. 12**). When Restylane and Radiesse are used in conjunction in the lower lid and midface complex, significant volume restoration can be achieved in a short period of time. Most recently, Sculptra (Sanofi-aventis US, Bridgewater, NJ, USA), a poly-L-lactic acid dermal filler, has been used for the midface by the authors' group, with comparable results (**Fig. 13**). A potential advantage of this treatment is the long-lasting effect of volume correction, but this must be tempered by the possibility of granuloma formation and foreign body reaction when placed directly in the periocular area. Careful observation and experience with Sculptra has emphasized the importance of thorough dilution of the powder with normal saline in a 6:1 or 8:1 concentration, as well as the delivery

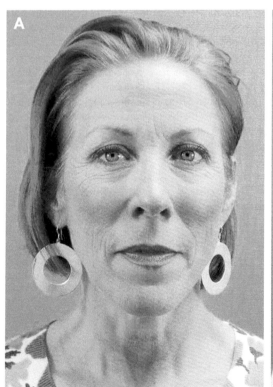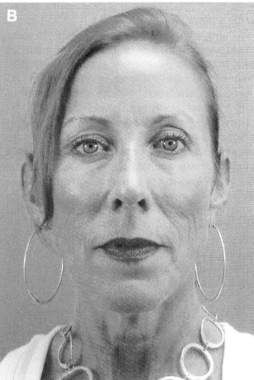

Fig. 13. (A) Preprocedure photograph of a woman, demonstrating loss of facial volume along the orbital rim and upper midface. (B) Postprocedure photograph after injection of 2 vials of Sculptra over a 3-month period, demonstrating volume restoration to the lower lid and midface.

of the product in a fan technique deep to the orbicularis muscle. The authors specifically avoid placement above the orbital rim and do not use a depot delivery technique.

SUMMARY

The authors think that complete rejuvenation of the middle third of the face can be achieved by addressing the aged lower lid and midface complex together as a single unit. These 2 regions are geographically confluent, and benefit from comprehensive analysis and simultaneous management.[1] Isolated surgical restoration of ptotic soft tissue and fat pads is as likely to be inadequate as volume restoration with dermal fillers alone, because most patients demonstrate combined gravitational descent and volume loss. By combining the subperiosteal midface lift with autologous lipotransfer, the authors' aesthetic results have significantly improved, and patients have benefited from reliable, long-lasting results. Dermal fillers such as Restylane, Radiesse, and Sculptra have a place in midfacial rejuvenation, particularly for those patients who are unwilling to undergo a surgical procedure and who desire the potential of a limited recovery phase. Even so, in the authors' experience autologous fat seems to provide more long-lasting results, allowing for a lower financial cost to the patient in the long term compared with sequential volume enhancement with dermal fillers on a periodic basis. In addition, the easily availability of additional fat permits the precise placement into volume-deficient areas without the concern of using a limited supply of a dermal filling agent.

There are many possible techniques and approaches to achieve effective midfacial rejuvenation. To ignore either the gravitational descent of the soft tissue and fat pads or the loss of facial volume will lead to consistent suboptimal results. The key is to perform a thorough facial analysis and establish the degree of ptotic descent and volume loss, so that a comprehensive treatment plan may be developed. The most natural results may occur by using a balanced approach that appropriately addresses the individual contributing components of midfacial aging.

REFERENCES

1. Lam SM, Chang EW, Rhee JS, et al. Perspective: rejuvenation of the periocular region: a unified approach to the eyebrow, midface, and eyelid complex. Ophthal Plast Reconstr Surg 2004; 20(1):1–9.
2. Defatta RJ, Williams EF 3rd. Evolution of midface rejuvenation. Arch Facial Plast Surg 2009;11(1):6–12.
3. Hamra ST. A study of the long-term effect of malar fat repositioning in face lift surgery: short-term success but long-term failure. Plast Reconstr Surg 2002;110(3):940–51.
4. Yousif NJ. Changes of the midface with age. Clin Plast Surg 1995;22(2):213–26.
5. Owsley JQ. Lifting the malar fat pad for correction of prominent nasolabial fold. Plast Reconstr Surg 1993; 91(3):463–74.
6. Ramirez OM. Endoscopic full facelift. Aesthetic Plast Surg 1994;18(4):363–71.
7. Williams EF, Lam SM. Upper and midfacial rejuvenation. In: Mikhli K, editor. Comprehensive facial rejuvenation. Philadelphia: Lippincott, Williams & Wilkins; 2003. p. 75–86.
8. Williams EF 3rd, Vargas H, Dahiya R, et al. Midfacial rejuvenation via a minimal-incision brow-lift approach: critical evaluation of a 5-year experience. Arch Facial Plast Surg 2003;5(6):470–8.
9. Hester TR, Codner MA, McCord CD, et al. Evolution of technique of the direct transblepharoplasty approach for the correction of lower lid and midfacial aging: maximizing results and minimizing complications in a 5 year experience. Plast Reconstr Surg 2000;105(1):393–406.
10. Coleman SR. Long-term survival of fat transplants: controlled demonstration. Aesthetic Plast Surg 1995;19(5):421–5.
11. Krishna S, Williams EF 3rd. Lipocontouring in conjunction with the minimal incision brow and subperiosteal midface lift: the next dimension in midface rejuvenation. Facial Plast Surg Clin North Am 2006; 14(3):221–8.
12. Pontius AT, Williams EF 3rd. The evolution of midface rejuvenation: combining the midface-lift and fat transfer. Arch Facial Plast Surg 2006;8(5):300–5.
13. DeFatta RJ, Williams EF 3rd. Fat transfer in conjunction with facial rejuvenation procedures. Facial Plast Surg Clin North Am 2008;16(4):383–90.

The Brow and Forehead in Periocular Rejuvenation

Laura Hetzler, MD, Jonathan Sykes, MD*

KEYWORDS

- Brow lift • Forehead lift • Brow ptosis
- Periocular rejuvenation

The periorbital region is often the first facial area to manifest signs of aging. The eyes may appear heavy or tired long before an individual experiences jowling or frank rhytids. The delicate anatomy of the eyes and periocular area make it more amenable to showing the signs of aging. Youthful patients have a full or volumized appearance to their skin, with notable subcutaneous fat. The thin skin of the upper and lower eyelids is nearly anatomically devoid of this subcutaneous fat and thus has less of a buffer to the early signs of aging.

In the past, the periocular and brow regions were inadequately addressed in facial rejuvenation surgery. The effect that the brow and forehead have on periocular and upper facial aging has not always been a priority. Contemporary surgeons have come to realize that one cannot improve the appearance of the upper eyelid if the brow is ptotic and continues to encroach upon the upper eyelid. If brow ptosis is present and not addressed, the periocular region continues to look heavy with a fatigued appearance.

The forehead, invariably linked with brow ptosis, has additional contributions to the aged appearance. The receding hairline in men or a prominent forehead in both sexes has an effect on overall facial appearance. Kinetic forehead rhytids caused by the hypertrophic corrugator, procerus, or frontalis muscles are natural repercussions of human expression. All these 3 muscles may cause brow asymmetry.

The entire face, having been broken down into aesthetic units, merits a thorough evaluation of symmetry and substance, which vary individually with patients. What does not vary, however, is the interaction and dependence of adjacent aesthetic units.

ANATOMY

The spatial position of an individual's brow is affected by the relative contribution of brow elevator versus brow depressor muscles. The frontalis muscle is the only elevator of the brow. This muscle ends anatomically at the superior temporal line.

There are, however, multiple depressor muscles, including the procerus, corrugator, depressor supercilii, and orbicularis oculi muscles. The procerus muscle is responsible for the horizontal glabellar rhytids, and the corrugator muscle for the vertical glabellar rhytids. The frontalis muscle is contained within the galea, which is a tendinous sheet that also envelops the occipitalis muscle. The galea is relatively inelastic and extends laterally to join with the temporoparietal fascia. This transition occurs at the temporal line. Although physically separated at the zygoma, the temporoparietal fascia is anatomically congruent with the superficial muscular aponeurotic system in the lower face below the zygomatic arch.

The orbicularis oculi is divided into 3 parts: preseptal, pretarsal, and orbital portions. This division is less of an anatomic designation and more of a functional division that aids the surgeon's decision for therapy as well as serves as a surgical landmark. The pretarsal and preseptal

Facial Plastic and Reconstructive Surgery, Department of Otolaryngology–Head and Neck Surgery, University of California, Davis, 2521 Stockton Boulevard, Suite 6206, Sacramento, CA 95817, USA
* Corresponding author.
E-mail address: jonathan.sykes@ucdmc.ucdavis.edu

Facial Plast Surg Clin N Am 18 (2010) 375–384
doi:10.1016/j.fsc.2010.04.002

components are self-explanatory, lying superficial to the tarsus and the orbital septum, respectively. These muscular subunits function somewhat involuntarily with blinking and are mechanical factors in the lacrimal pump system. The orbital portion of the orbicularis oculi functions in squinting and is more of a cause for dynamic rhytids, including the crow's feet. This orbital portion is implicated in brow ptosis, medially and laterally.

The skin of the forehead is thick and is densely adhered to the underlying subcutaneous tissue. Deep to the subcutaneous tissue is the previously mentioned galea aponeurosis containing the frontalis muscles anteriorly and the occipitalis muscle posteriorly. The galea is separated from the periosteum by loose connective tissue. The periosteum is contiguous laterally with temporalis muscle fascia at the temporal line. The periosteum of the forehead has a confluence with the orbital septum at the superior orbital rim. This dense fascia condensation is called the arcus marginalis (**Fig. 1**). It is imperative that these decussating fibers be released for adequate and enduring brow-lift results.

PREOPERATIVE EVALUATION

In the preoperative evaluation, it is the surgeon's responsibility to point out the asymmetries in brow position and the importance of the brow and its effect on the upper eyelid. The surgeon must also communicate why correcting excess lid skin and fat herniation fails in improving appearance if the ptotic brow is not addressed.

Ideal brow position varies between gender and race. Men tend to have a heavier, thicker brow, with little arc present. The brow in men lies approximately at the level of the superior orbital rim. The brow in women is more refined. In women, the brow is club shaped medially and tapers laterally.

The medial border of the brow is on a vertical line with the alar-facial crease. The lateral end of the brow lies on a line drawn from the alar-facial crease tangent to the lateral canthus. The medial and lateral ends of the brow are on the same horizontal plane. The highest arch of the brow in women is ideally at the lateral limbus or just lateral to it. Ideally, the brow in women should lie just above the superior orbital rim (**Fig. 2**).[1]

It is important for the patient to be in complete repose during evaluation. Often, patients with brow ptosis compensate by tonic contraction of the frontalis muscle, which may result in headaches as well as horizontal forehead rhytids. To achieve full repose, it may be beneficial to ask patients to close their eyes, focus on relaxing the forehead, and gently open their eyes for a more precise analysis of brow position.

McKinney and colleagues[2] described certain quantitative measurements to aid in selection of the appropriate lifting technique. The investigators used measurements in a vertical plane from mid-pupil to the top of the eyebrow and up to the hairline to indicate which procedures and approaches should be used for brow lifting. The investigators prefer to use a more individualized approach for

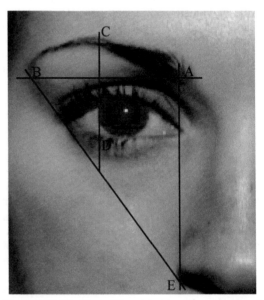

Fig. 2. Ideal brow position in a woman. The lateral brow lies at or above the medial brow (AB). The medial brow begins along a vertical line drawn from the nasal ala (AE). The brow peaks at the lateral limbus of the iris (CD). The lateral brow extends to a line drawn through the lateral canthus to the ala (BE). (*Modified from* Gunter JP, Antrobus SD. Aesthetic analysis of the eyebrows. Plast Reconstr Surg 1997;99(7):1808–16; with permission.)

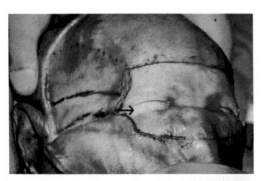

Fig. 1. The cadaver image illustrates the arcus marginalis (*black arrow*) as the reflection of periosteum from the forehead into the orbit as it becomes the orbital septum.

brow and periocular evaluation, focusing on specific anatomic landmarks.

Eyelid Ptosis

It is important to note if a patient has underlying eyelid ptosis on one or both sides, which is best determined by assessing the marginal reflex distance (MRD) 1. MRD-1 is the noted distance between pupillary light reflex and the margin of the upper lid; a distance of 3.5 to 5 mm is normal. The upper lid itself should lie just below the superior limbus by approximately 1 to 1.5 mm. The MRD-2 is the distance, measured again in primary gaze, between the pupillary light reflex and lower lid margin; a distance of greater than 5 mm is adequate.

Levator Function

Levator function must also be recorded when evaluating brow ptosis. This evaluation is performed by holding the brow in position (nullifying the effect of the frontalis muscle) and requesting the patient to first look down and then up. The difference between the eyelid position looking downward and then upward is the levator function (**Fig. 3**). If a measurement of less than 4 mm is found

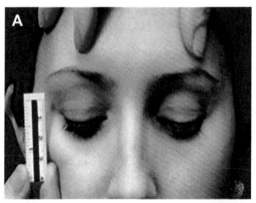
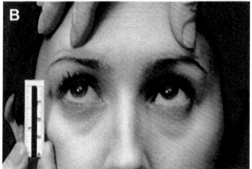

Fig. 3. (A, B) Frontal image showing how to assess the function of the levator palpebrae superioris before surgical intervention.

between maximum downgaze and maximum upgaze, the levator function is deemed as poor; a movement of 5 to 7 mm is fair, 8 to 15 mm is good, and more than 15 mm is normal (**Table 1**).

Upper Lid

Upper lid evaluation is to be performed in conjunction with brow evaluation. An attenuated skin excision is appropriate after brow elevation to avoid excessive lagophthalmos. Dermatochalasia is the general term used for presence of excessive skin and its laxity associated with aging as well as fat herniation. Blepharochalasis is a rare occurrence of unknown cause that occurs typically in women and is manifest by edema, causing decreased elasticity and notable atrophic changes.

Forehead

The forehead itself may mandate the appropriate brow procedure. Deep forehead rhytids with a high hairline make midforehead lift a reasonable approach.

Patient Health

The patient's health may also play a role in preoperative decisions. Unhealthy patients who are not suited for longer surgeries or general anesthesia may preclude more extensive procedures and elect a direct brow approach.

PREOPERATIVE CONSIDERATIONS

The authors routinely use botulinum toxin before most brow lifts in the cosmetic setting. The use of botulinum toxin before brow lifting eliminates the function of the brow depressors, including the corrugator, procerus, and orbicularis oculi muscles (**Fig. 4**). The absence of the persistent depressor function promotes longevity of the brow lift as well as allows readherance of the forehead flap to the underlying cranium. This readherance has been shown to occur within 1 week after surgery.[3] Botulinum toxin injection is performed at

Table 1 Range of levator palpebrae superioris function	
Levator Muscle Excursion (mm)	Functional Classification
<4	Poor
5–7	Fair
8–15	Good
>15	Normal

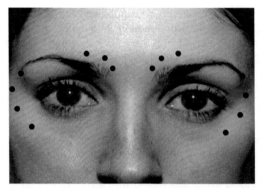

Fig. 4. Sites for preoperative botulinum toxin injection to promote longevity of brow lift and ideal healing.

least 10 days preoperatively to allow adequate neurotoxin effect.

The position of the medial and lateral brow needs to be evaluated separately. The lateral brow often warrants more vigorous elevation, whereas the medial brow is best approached conservatively and should not be overly elevated. The authors are routinely more cautious with medial release to avoid an overly elevated medial brow and a surprised appearance.

TECHNIQUES IN BROW LIFTING AND FOREHEAD REJUVENATION
Surgical Techniques

Transblepharoplasty browpexy
The benefit of the transblepharoplasty approach is that the incisions are hidden within a natural skin crease. The disadvantages of this approach are that the amount of brow elevation to be achieved is limited and there may be an increased risk of supraorbital nerve injury and associated numbness. Anchoring sutures are placed from the brow soft tissues to the periosteum above the level of the supraorbital rim. Inadvertent stretching of the incision with dissection and fixation may damage incisional skin, leading to poor scarring. The transblepharoplasty approach allows less dissection, causing less bruising and postoperative discomfort than other methods of addressing brow ptosis.

Direct approach
Direct brow lifting may be useful in patients unfit for a more extensive surgery, when functional improvement is the main objective. The direct brow lift may be performed under local anesthesia, with or without sedation. Although the dissection required is minimal, there is an increased risk of brow hair loss because of transection of hair follicles.

An incision is marked along the superior edge of the brow along its full length. This mark is placed just within the most superior rows of the brow hairs. Injection of 1% xylocaine with 1:100,000 epinephrine is used and allowed to take effect for at least 10 minutes. A scalpel is then used to make an incision parallel to the hair follicles to avoid transection of the follicles and postoperative alopecia. The brow is then pulled superiorly with a skin hook to the appropriate level of elevation and the skin is marked. This procedure is performed multiple times along the length of the brow to create a proposed amount of skin to be excised. Care is taken to avoid damage to the supraorbital nerves and vessels, which may entail performing a more superficial incision medially and a more full thickness excision laterally to include muscle.

Closure is performed in 3 layers:

1. Fixation sutures, using a permanent monofilament such as Prolene, are performed from the brow soft tissues to the periosteum of the frontal bone at a level of appropriate elevation.
2. Absorbable buried deep sutures are placed to alleviate any tension on the closure. These sutures should extend to the deep dermis.
3. The skin may then be closed in such a fashion to maximize eversion with a nonabsorbable monofilament suture. This closure could include alternating simple interrupted and vertical mattress sutures or running horizontal mattress sutures. Care must be taken not to create too much of an arch in men resulting in feminization of the brow.

The direct approach described is still in use by some surgeons but is not used in the senior author's (JS) practice.

Midforehead approach
The midforehead approach is excellent at achieving a precise brow lift with minimal dissection. The approach is beneficial particularly in patients with obvious forehead rhytids and high hairlines and also in those with unilateral cranial nerve VII paralysis. The midforehead approach is particularly effective in men because the scar hides nicely within the horizontal furrows. This approach is in contrast to a direct brow incision, which may require makeup for camouflage.[4]

Incisions can be placed in horizontal forehead creases, preferably not at the same level on each side. If creases are chosen at the same level, they should not extend across midline to create the appearance of a complete linear scar (**Fig. 5A**).

The skin to be excised is marked before injecting local anesthetic. Midforehead brow lifting may be performed under general anesthesia or

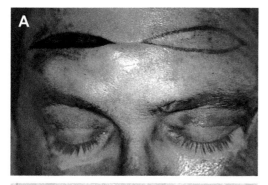

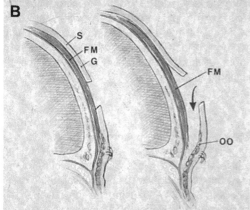

Fig. 5. (A) Placement of midforehead brow-lift incision. (B) The author's preferred dissection plane in the subcutaneous plane. FM, frontalis muscle; G, galea; oo, orbicularisoculi; S, skin.

monitored intravenous sedation. The fusiform incisions are made at the level of the previously marked furrow and carried into the immediate subcutaneous tissue. Undermining is performed in the subcutaneous, supramuscular plane (see **Fig. 5B**).

The extent of dissection is from the incision superiorly to the level of the brow inferiorly. If the glabellar rhytids are to be addressed with either lysis or resection of the brow depressors, the subperiosteal plane may be entered medially, with care taken to avoid injury to the supraorbital neurovascular bundle. Subperiosteal dissection may be extended laterally for release of the arcus marginalis. Release of the arcus is usually not necessary for this approach to achieve adequate lifting and is rarely performed by the senior author. The skin is then redraped superiorly to a level providing adequate brow elevation.

Excess skin is excised accordingly to allow for brow elevation. The superior skin edge must be undermined to allow for skin eversion during closure. Fixation is performed using a 4-0 permanent monofilament such as Prolene (Ethicon, Somerville, NJ, USA), securing the soft tissues of the brow and orbicularis oculi muscle to the periosteum superiorly. Deeply buried dermal sutures may be required to remove any tension in closure, and the skin is closed as in the direct brow lift. One may consider beveling the skin incision away from the skin resection to allow for adequate skin eversion. Beveling cannot be performed well in the direct brow lift because the incision must follow the hair follicles.

McKinney and colleagues[2] discuss the merits of using the midforehead technique particularly in men. The scar of a midforehead lift would be more visible in a younger patient, as would the scar of a direct brow lift, making these approaches preferable for rehabilitative rather than cosmetic uses.

Pretrichial approach

The pretrichial approach to brow lifting is ideal in patients with a high hairline. The incision is marked 2 mm posterior to the hairline centrally and within the temporal hair laterally, as seen in **Fig. 6**. The area is injected with xylocaine 1% with 1:100,000 epinephrine at the incision and along the entire forehead. A scalpel is used to make a trichophyllic incision with the bevel anteriorly to allow the hair follicles of the superior flap to grow through the inferior skin to aid in scar camouflage (see **Fig. 6**). The incision is advanced to the subgaleal

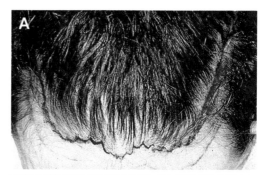

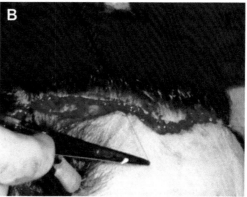

Fig. 6. (A) Intraoperative photograph of a trichophyllic incision for a trichophytic brow lift and (B) closure.

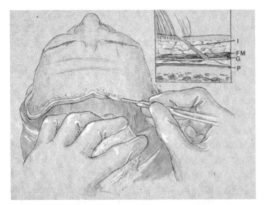

Fig. 7. The trichophytic brow-lift setup with surgeon at the head of the bead. Inset demonstrates the appropriate subgaleal plane. FM, frontalis muscle; G, galea; I, incision; P, periostium.

plane and then elevated down to approximately 3 to 4 cm above the supraorbital rim (**Fig. 7**). At this point, the periosteum is incised and elevated down to the nasal bones, with care taken not to injure the supraorbital and supratrochlear neurovascular bundles.

The lateral incision shifts into the temporal hair and extends down through the temporoparietal fascia onto the superficial layer of deep temporal fascia overlying the temporalis muscle. The dissection plane proceeds between the temporoparietal fascia containing the frontal branch of the facial nerve and on top of the superficial layer of the deep temporal fascia. Care is taken to release the arcus marginalis without injuring the supraorbital neurovascular bundle, which allows adequate release of the lateral brow.

The flap may then be secured with suture alone; suture with bone bridge, either free hand or Bone Bridge System (Medtronic Xomed, Jacksonville, FL, USA); ENDOTINE fixation device (Coapt Systems, Inc, Palo Alto, CA, USA); or tissue adhesives.

In the pretrichial brow lift, the authors prefer excision and closure of the galea with absorbable monofilament suture. Following adequate skin excision, the incision is closed with staples for the temporal hair-baring region and with 5-0 or 6-0 running locking nonabsorbable monofilament suture for the more central incision just within the hairline (**Fig. 8**).

Coronal approach

The coronal incision is typically just anterior to the vertex in a wavy line pattern and must always be made parallel to the hair follicles to avoid postoperative alopecia. Exposure and dissection planes are within the subgaleal plane, similar to the pretrichial dissection. When using the coronal approach for brow lifting, fixation and closure is performed identically to the pretrichial lift.[5] The disadvantages of this approach are elevation of the hairline and troublesome numbness as well as a risk for alopecia and skin necrosis. The coronal approach

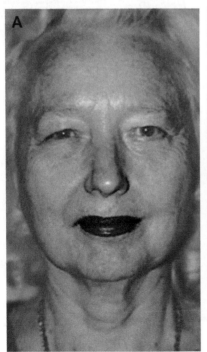

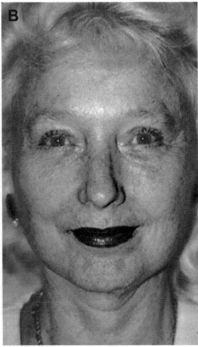

Fig. 8. Preoperative (*A*) and postoperative (*B*) photographs of a trichophytic brow lift.

is ideal for patients with a lower hairline without significant thinning of vertex hair. In men with male pattern baldness, the incision can be made further posteriorly on the vertex to allow camouflage of the incision.

It is generally accepted that the more distant the surgical incision is from the brow the more skin excision is necessary. More skin must be excised for the desired level of brow elevation using a coronal approach compared with the pretrichial incision. In the hairline incision, the ratio of the amount of skin incision to the brow lift is 1:5, whereas in the coronal approach it is closer to 2:1.[5]

Endoscopic approach

The endoscopic approach to brow lifting allows for minimal, well-concealed incisions that preserve scalp and forehead sensation. There is minimal blood loss and preservation of a well-vascularized soft-tissue flap. The endoscopic brow lift allows for earlier resolution of soft tissue edema and minimal change in the length of the forehead.

Initially, 3 incisions are made: 1 in the midline and 2 bilaterally at the level of the lateral brow in line with the proposed vector of suspension. The incisions are made just behind the hairline and are roughly 1- to 1.5-cm long. The initial 3 incisions are made through all layers of the scalp. The entire forehead periosteum is elevated from the hairline to approximately 2 cm above the orbital rim. Care must be taken not to damage the periosteum because it may impair visualization and durability of resuspension.

At this point, a 30° endoscope with a protective sheath is introduced near the supraorbital rim for further elevation of the flap. The supraorbital neurovascular bundle should be directly visualized and preserved with careful dissection. Of note, 10% of the population have the nerve and vessels exiting through a true foramen, rather than a notch. At this point, resection or lysis of the corrugator superciliary muscle may be performed. Some investigators also perform a radial myotomy of the orbicularis oculi muscle deep to the brow. Lateral release of the periosteum is performed at the arcus marginalis at the level of the orbital rim (**Fig. 9**).

The 2 temporal incisions are made overlying the temporalis muscle. The position of these incisions corresponds to the vector of pull needed for the desired brow position. Again, beveling is performed for follicle preservation. The incision is carried down through skin, subcutaneous tissue, and temporoparietal fascia. The dissection plane proceeds deep to the temporoparietal fascia, just on top of the superficial layer of deep temporal fascia overlying the temporalis muscle extending down to the level of the lateral canthus. Dissection

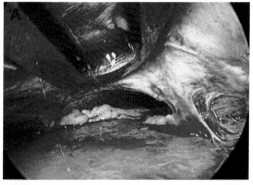
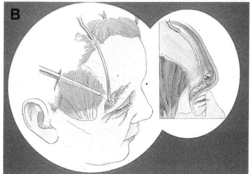

Fig. 9. (*A*) Intraoperative photograph of arcus marginalis release. (*B*) Release of arcus marginalis under direct endoscopic visualization.

may be performed under direct visualization (**Fig. 10**). The lateral subgaleal and medial subperiosteal planes of dissection are connected by dividing the conjoint tendon at the superior temporal line. The conjoint tendon connects the superficial and deep layers of temporalis fascia and their medial extension, the pericranium, as well as the junction of the temporoparietal fascia laterally and the galea medially (**Fig. 11**). The

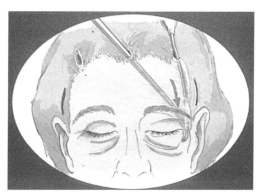

Fig. 10. Standard 5 incisions used in an endoscopic brow lifting, with midline port used for endoscope insertion.

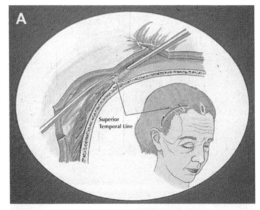

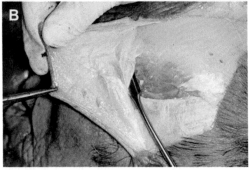

Fig. 11. (*A*) Release of the conjoint tendon connecting the lateral subgaleal plane and the medial subperiosteal plane at the superior temporal line. (*B*) Left-sided conjoint tendon at the superior temporal line in a cadaver.

sentinel vein may be visualized laterally and is a marker for the frontal branch of the facial nerve. This vein is an extension of the internal maxillary vein and should be preserved. Extension of this

dissection is performed inferiorly to the orbital rim to ensure full release of the arcus marginalis.

After complete elevation and release of the brow-forehead complex, suspension is performed bilaterally in the temporal and lateral brow regions. The temporal area is first suspended. The temporoparietal fascia is suspended to the deep temporal fascia with a 2-0 monofilament absorbable suture.

Resuspension of the brow and forehead skin is performed next at the incisions made in line with lateral brow. The senior author prefers a bone bridge method using a monofilament absorbable suture, such as 2-0 polydioxanone. A bone tunnel may be performed free hand as well as with the Bone Bridge System (**Fig. 12**). Tissue adhesives, the ENDOTINE fixation device, and microscrews may also be used (**Figs. 13** and **14**). Brodner and colleagues,[3] in their study with Australian white rabbits, showed that periosteal readherence occurs within 1 week after brow lift, therefore negating the need for long-term resuspension.

COMPLICATIONS

Complications of brow lift procedures vary with the approach and incision used.

Visible Scars

Obviously, the most glaring complications of direct and midforehead lift are visible scars.

Hematoma

As with any surgery, all brow-lift approaches have the risk of hematomas.

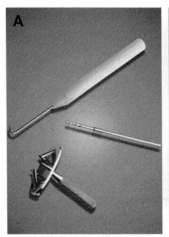

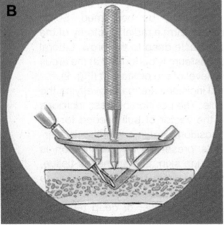

Fig. 12. Bone Bridge System.

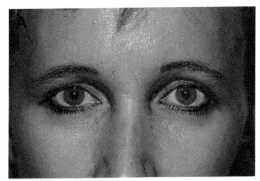

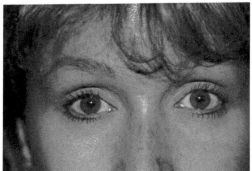

Fig. 13. Preoperative (*A*) and postoperative (*B*) frontal photographs of an endoscopic brow lift. Note the improved position of the lateral brow.

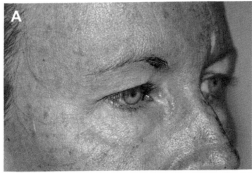

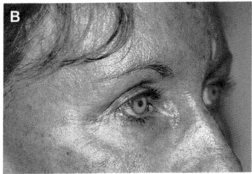

Fig. 14. Preoperative (*A*) and postoperative (*B*) right-sided oblique photographs of an endoscopic brow lift. Note the improved position of the lateral brow. This patient also benefited from an upper and lower blepharoplasty.

Loss of Sensation

The pretrichial and the coronal approaches are associated with significant transient sensory anesthesia of the scalp and forehead. Sensation typically returns over the course of months, with improvements in sensation starting nearer the brow and extending toward the vertex, typically with full return of sensation by 12 months.

Alopecia

Alopecia can also occur from either poorly created or poorly closed incisions, including inappropriate wound tension. Peri-incisional alopecia can lead to what appears to be a widened scar.

Nerve Damage

Damage to the frontal branch of the facial nerve can occur.

Brow Asymmetry

Brow asymmetry can result from failure to elevate either brow adequately. Failure to achieve adequate elevation is likely the result of unsuccessful release of the orbital rim tissues. Adverse hairline alteration can hopefully be avoided with appropriate choice of approach.

ADJUNCT PROCEDURES

During a brow lift, many have promoted myotomies and myectomies of the corrugator and procerus complex as well as orbicularis and frontalis. This procedure has been described in the literature as early as the 1970s.[6] However, the permanent benefit of myotomies has been questioned at times. The procedure may also have some disadvantages, such as widening of the space between the medial brows and, in the case of a frontal myotomy, depression of the brow.

Neurotoxins such as botulinum toxin have been helpful in prolonging a brow lift and may be used as an adjunct preoperatively. Neurotoxins also have the additional benefit of deterring future rhytids.

As with any facial rejuvenation surgery, attention to the soft tissue envelope is imperative. The forehead often displays a patient's history of sun exposure and subsequent discoloration and elastosis. Medical or topical adjuncts may be used to improve the appearance and quality of the skin and thus further improve the surgical result.

Table 2
Dissection planes in the medial and temporal regions and the type of fixations for various approaches of brow lifting

Approach	Midline Plane	Lateral Plane (Temporal)	Fixation
Direct	Subcutaneous	N/A	Soft tissue to soft tissue
Midforehead	Subcutaneous[a]	N/A	Soft tissue to soft tissue
Pretrichial	Subgaleal	Subgaleal	Soft tissue to soft tissue
Coronal	Subgaleal	Subgaleal	Soft tissue to soft tissue
Endoscopic[b]	Subperiosteal	Subgaleal	Soft tissue to bone bridge[c]

Abbreviation: N/A, not applicable.
[a] Some surgeons prefer to use a subperiosteal dissection also.
[b] Medial and temporal planes are joined by releasing conjoint tendon.
[c] Authors prefer bone bridge method.

SUMMARY

Evaluation of the periocular region is paramount when performing rejuvenation of the upper face. Recognition of the brow as an integral contributor to periocular appearance improves and prolongs results from facial rejuvenation surgery. The approach to the brow and forehead must be chosen on an individual basis, with particular attention given to a person's hairline and hair recession patterns, alopecia, forehead length, relative need for elevation between the medial and lateral brow, functional versus cosmetic reasons for pursuing a brow lift, forehead skin and rhytids, and the patient's goals and expectations. The approaches discussed require in-depth knowledge of complex forehead and temporal anatomy to navigate the planes and important neurovascular structures safely **(Table 2)**.

REFERENCES

1. Gunter JP, Antrobus SD. Aesthetic analysis of the eyebrows. Plast Reconstr Surg 1997;99:1808–16.
2. McKinney P, Mossie RD, Zukowski ML. Criteria for the forehead lift. Aesthetic Plast Surg 1991;15:141.
3. Brodner DC, Downs JC, Graham HD. Periosteal re-adherence after browlift in the New Zealand white rabbit. Arch Facial Plast Surg 2002;4: 247–51.
4. Rafferty FM, Goode RL, Abramson NR. The brow lift operation in a man. Arch Otolaryngol 1978; 104:69–71.
5. Leach J. Browlifting. Operat Tech Otolaryngol Head Neck Surg 2007;18:162–5.
6. Pitanguy I. Section of the frontalis-procerus-corrugator aponeurosis in the correction of frontal and glabellar wrinkles. Ann Plast Surg 1979; 2(5):422–7.

Autologous Fat and Fillers in Periocular Rejuvenation

Edward D. Buckingham, MD[a],*, Bradford Bader, MD[b],
Stephen P. Smith, MD[b]

KEYWORDS

- Facial aging • Hyaluronic acid • Calcium hydroxylapatite
- Autologous fat

Volume loss has increasingly been recognized as an important aspect of facial aging. This is especially true of the periocular region. Restoration of this lost volume can be achieved through placement of syringe-based fillers, autologous fat, or implants. This article discusses the use of syringe-based fillers (hyaluronic acid, calcium hydroxylapatite) and autologous fat to rejuvenate the periorbital region.

The periorbital complex consists of the brow, superior orbital rim, upper eyelid, lateral canthus, lower eyelid, inferior orbital rim, and upper cheek. The most important of these in the aging process of volume loss is the interface between the lower eyelid and upper cheek or midface. Systematic aging begins throughout the periorbital complex beginning in the patient's mid-to-late 30s.[1] The extent and rapidity of periorbital aging varies between individuals and is strongly dependent on the relationships between the bony orbit, globe, and malar complex. The periorbital area ages at a faster pace and earlier in life with a negative vector midface, much as the jaw line and neck age earlier in people with microgenia and a short thyromental distance (**Fig. 1**). Some individuals even display "lower eyelid bags" in youth; these bags appear early because of the negative vector produced by the deficient anterior projection of the inferior orbital rim in relation to the globe.

YOUTH

The youthful upper periorbital complex consists of a brow that is full over its entire height, being propped up by the volume of the brow fat pad. Entire articles have been written and rewritten about the normal aesthetic height of the brow.[2] The authors are well aware of these aesthetic norms but maintain that patients differ tremendously regarding their natural brow height. They ask their patients routinely about their brow position in youth and strive to restore this relationship, only changing natural brow position after careful consideration. Comparing photos in the latest fashion magazine shows many examples of models, all of whom are exquisitely attractive, with significantly differing relationships between the brow and superior orbital rim (**Fig. 2**). The upper eyelid also shows a variable fullness between patients; all may be considered youthful and attractive. Some individuals have significant tarsal show with a deep superior orbital sulcus, a high lid crease, and very little dermatochalasia. Others have very little tarsal show with a more prominent orbital fat component and therefore, a much fuller-appearing upper eyelid and a tendency toward greater dermatochalasia. In the authors' opinion, the restoration of the youthful upper eyelid and brow complex must be tailored to each patient's unique characteristics and must

Disclosures: Edward Buckingham is a promotional speaker for Medicis.
[a] Buckingham Center for Facial Plastic Surgery, 102 Westlake Drive, Suite 104, Austin, TX 78746, USA
[b] Division of Facial Plastic and Reconstructive Surgery, Department of Otolaryngology-Head and Neck Surgery, The Ohio State University Medical Center, 410 West 10th Avenue, Columbus, OH 43210, USA
* Corresponding author.
E-mail address: edbuckin@yahoo.com

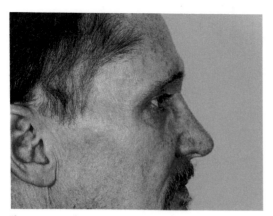

Fig. 1. Lateral view of male patient demonstrating negative vector association between globe and inferior orbital rim.

strive toward the restoration of youthfulness and not an ideal appearance based on the biases of the surgeon. Some rejuvenation of the upper eyelid complex relies on surgical lifting procedures that are beyond the scope of this article. However, restoration of the upper periorbital volume is addressed.

The youthful lower eyelid complex revolves around the appearance of a short lower eyelid, or rather, a superiorly placed and full upper cheek. The lower eyelid cheek interface should be at the lower tarsal border and flow into a full convex upper anterior cheek. This natural convex fullness results from the quantity of the lower eyelid suborbicularis oculi fat or SOOF and also depends heavily on inferior orbital rim projection (**Fig. 3**). The youthful lower eyelid must also lack pseudoherniation of orbital fat. The cheek skin should be smooth over the underlying fat and the malar cheek fat pad should be shaped as a teardrop, with the rounded leading edge of the tear

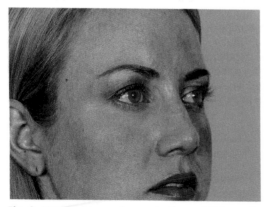

Fig. 2. Young woman demonstrating a full brow fat pad with a soft superior orbital rim and plump support for the brow.

inferior-medial and tapering laterally over the anterior aspect of the zygomatic arch. The inferior aspect of this teardrop should create a subtle shadow in its interface with the buccal region that parallels that of the jaw line (**Fig. 4**). These features lead to the overall appearance of the heart-shaped face of youth.

AGING

Aging is the culmination of a multifactorial process that includes the actions of gravity, volume loss, and skin changes due to intrinsic and extrinsic factors. Volume loss in the periorbital area leads to exposure of harsh bony contours and the creation of shadows indicating aging. In the superior rim, this also leads to an apparent descent of the brow. As volume is lost over the bony orbital rim, the support for the soft tissue brow is lost. This effectively raises the position of the bony rim, which is now harsh and skeletonized, and leads to an apparent drop in brow height because the hair-bearing eyebrow now rests in a lower position relative to the superior orbital rim. This volumetric contribution to brow aging is not the only component. Forehead, brow, and upper eyelid aging is a complex process with a gravitational contribution that may benefit from surgical lifting procedures; however, volume is an important consideration. Photos of the patient when young are a valuable tool in assessing the relative contributions of different factors in periorbital aging, thus assisting the surgeon in the appropriate selection of rejuvenation techniques.

Lower periorbital/cheek aging is most significantly influenced by volume-related changes. With time, the heart-shaped youthful face gives way to the more rectangular face of age. Some of this is due to the development of jowling and lower facial aging, which is beyond the scope of this discussion. The loss of volume in the lower eyelid/cheek complex, however, is a key contributor to the rectangular face. Additionally, volume loss allows the appearance of shadows, as tissues fall and become tethered by various retaining ligaments. Double contours arise in the lower eyelid and cheek, with exposed orbital fat creating a bulge, the exposed bony orbital rim creating a hollow, malar mound bulge, and malar septum hollow (**Fig. 5**). The lower eyelid gains apparent length in this process. Pseudoherniation of lower eyelid orbital fat combined with loss of orbital rim volume leads to lengthening of the lower lid height and inferior placement of the lower eyelid cheek junction. This is the orbital groove/tear trough deformity. Below this, the malar mound and malar septum create a second double contour in the

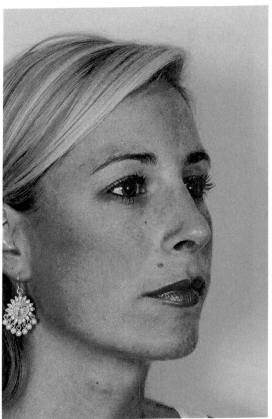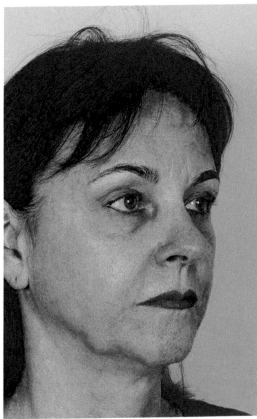

Fig. 3. Youthful lower eyelid complex with short-appearing lower eyelid and smooth transition between the lower eyelid and cheek compared with typical aged lower eyelid cheek complex with a long-appearing lower eyelid and orbital groove.

cheek region. Restoration of youth combines removal of orbital fat pseudoherniation, if indicated, and placement of volume into the orbital groove/tear trough and cheek region to restore the single convexity of the cheek and raise the cheek eyelid junction, thereby shortening the apparent lower lid height.

PATIENT ASSESSMENT

Although people are becoming more educated about volume loss as a cause of their facial aging, patients rarely present for consultation requesting a fat transfer. Patients express concern that they appear tired or that they have persistent dark circles under their eyes. A detailed assessment is necessary to determine the cause of their concerns and what part of this is due to volume loss. Review of patient photographs from their youth is helpful, but if these are not available, pointed questions about eyelid appearance and brow height can help differentiate between age-related changes and normal anatomic variation.

A detailed history and physical examination is indicated; however, the authors limit discussion to the key factors related to volume replacement. Much of forehead and upper eyelid rejuvenation relies on incisional techniques. However, brow position and brow fat quantity should be assessed. In many instances, the brow height is adequate, and adding volume alone to the superior orbital rim will restore a youthful appearance. A hollow superior orbital sulcus may also be restored with volume, although this is an advanced technique and careful patient consultation should take place regarding the likelihood of contour irregularities. The authors address the hollow superior orbital sulcus with a patient only if it is a specific concern and usually offer intervention only if it is due to previous surgical misadventures and not a natural occurrence. The mainstay of patient assessment for volume replacement involves the lower eyelid and cheek.

Assessment of the lower eyelid and cheek begins with determining if orbital fat pseudoherniation requires addressing. This determination is

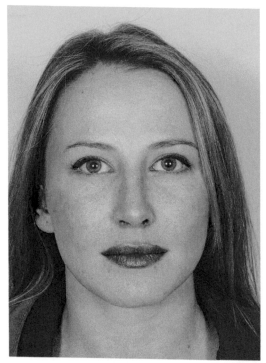

Fig. 4. Youthful female with full malar volume demonstrating the teardrop configuration of the cheek and the subtle shadow of the inframalar area that parallels the jaw line.

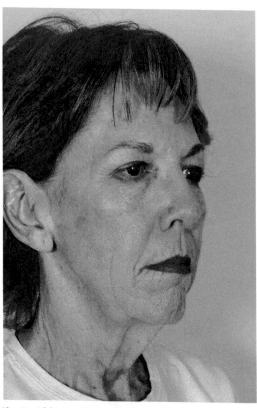

Fig. 5. Oblique photo of a severely aged lower eyelid cheek complex demonstrating the long-appearing lower eyelid with an orbital groove, the hollow, volume deficient cheek with a malar groove, and double contour of the lower eyelid and cheek.

made by evaluating the patient in oblique and lateral views. If the orbital fat protrudes anterior, beyond the surgeon's perception of a natural convex cheek eyelid interface, a blepharoplasty should be considered (**Fig. 6**). This usually involves only the medial and middle fat compartments because the lateral fat compartment less commonly protrudes beyond the desired convex line. A transconjunctival technique is used with minimal exposure because the tissue planes need to be preserved over the orbital rim for concurrent fat grafting. An assessment of overall midface volume and position is also performed, noting a negative vector midface (prominent eyes), the presence of a malar groove, malar septum, and malar mound, especially if early festooning is present. Assessment of the lower cheek is also made, including buccal hollowing and perioral volume loss. Once assessments of the relative contributions of volume loss have been made, a conversation with the patient may begin regarding intervention.

Patients presenting earlier in the aging process who lack significant volume loss or a bony negative vector and who do not require a lower eyelid blepharoplasty are candidates for office-based volume replacement with syringe-based fillers or surgical treatment with autologous fat. As patients develop more severe volume loss that would require multiple syringes of filling material to achieve results, the financial outlay on the material makes fat grafting a better option. Additionally, fat has the advantages of being durable with long-term graft survival. Each option, including its longevity, down-time, results, and cost, are discussed with patients, following which they can select the procedure that best fits their wishes.

HYALURONIC ACID TECHNIQUE

Hyaluronic acid (HA; Restylane, Perlane, Juvederm, etc) is used for patients who do not have a severe degree of aging or who have a greater degree of aging but wish to avoid the expense or recovery associated with more invasive procedures.[3–8] The HA is mixed with 0.2 mL of 2% Xylocaine with 1:100,000 units of epinephrine using a sterile stainless steel double Luer-Lok coupling. For the brow, no other anesthesia is used. For the lower eyelid and cheek, a small amount of

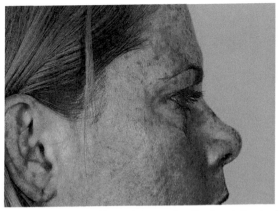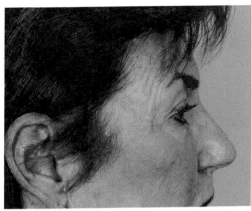

Fig. 6. Comparison of lateral views of patient on left who lacks steatoblepharon and underwent only a fat transfer and patient on right with a sufficient steatoblepharon to warrant a transconjunctival blepharoplasty and fat transfer.

1% Xylocaine without epinephrine is place through an intraoral route at the infraorbital nerve foramen. Brow injection is performed by palpating the reflection of the supraorbital rim with the index finger and thumb of the nondominant hand. A direct injection deep to the orbicularis muscle and superficial to the periosteum is performed in small aliquots until brow fullness is restored. Care is taken to avoid the supraorbital neurovascular bundle. Injection is usually lateral to this landmark. For the lower eyelid orbital groove/tear trough, the area to be injected is first marked out with a fine-tip surgical marking pen. The premixed HA is then injected with a 31-gauge needle beginning medially. Care is taken at the medial injection point to avoid the angular vein, and aspiration is performed before injection. The material is placed just superficial to the periosteum in small aliquots. Injection then progresses laterally, placing more material adjacent to the last injection until a confluence of the smaller injections occurs. Gentle massage can be performed to manipulate the material into a smooth configuration (**Fig. 7**). Once the initial deep injection is complete, further material is added just deep to or within the orbicularis muscle to further refine the area. On the second pass, the area is anesthetized from the local anesthetic placed during the first pass. This allows further refinement to be precisely performed with no patient discomfort. Observation is made of the superficial veins of the lower lid, which are avoided. If any bleeding occurs, pressure with a Q-tip or gauze is immediately performed to minimize bruising and prevent an accumulation of blood, which makes assessment of correction difficult. The goal is to achieve barely full to slight undercorrection. The authors err on the side of undercorrection; a ridge of filler may

be visible with any degree of overcorrection (**Fig. 8**).

Lower eyelid filler always creates small pinpoint areas of ecchymosis, which usually resolve within 3 to 5 days and can be easily covered with makeup. More significant bruising occasionally occurs but can usually be avoided by having the patient eliminate any blood-thinning medication in advance. The most common complication is undercorrection, which may be touched up 2 to 4 weeks after the initial treatment. Patients are told that a small touch-up may be required to achieve optimal results. Most patients are satisfied with one treatment and most do not seek refinement. Small contour irregularities can usually be manipulated with gentle massage and will resolve. More significant overcorrection should be avoided, but in the most severe cases, hyaluronidase may be used in small quantities to enzymatically degrade the product. However, this usually leads to near-complete return to the pretreatment appearance.

CALCIUM HYDROXYLAPATITE TECHNIQUE

Radiesse (Bioform Medical Inc, Franksville, WI, USA) is a synthetic injectable implant composed of smooth calcium hydroxylapatite (CaHA) microspheres (diameter of 25–45 μm) suspended in a sodium carboxymethylcellulose gel carrier. Radiesse is Food and Drug Administration (FDA)-approved for the correction of moderate-to-severe facial folds and wrinkles, such as nasolabial folds, and for the correction of signs of facial lipoatrophy in HIV-positive patients. There are also FDA clearances for oral/maxillofacial defects, vocal fold augmentation, and radiographic tissue marking. Radiesse does not contain any animal

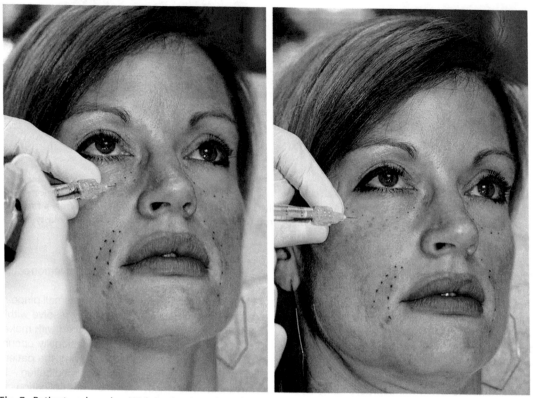

Fig. 7. Patient undergoing HA injection into the orbital groove. The area for injection has been marked out. The photo on the left demonstrates the medial groove being injected and on the right, nearing completion of the right lower eyelid.

products, and skin testing is not required before use. Upon injection, it initially acts as a filler. It is easily malleable, can be used to shape and contour large areas of the face, and provides results patients can appreciate immediately. Once injected, the CaHA microspheres are slowly degraded by the body and stimulate neocollagenesis. Most authors report a treatment effect that lasts 6 to 12 months (**Fig. 9**).[9,10]

For treatment, the patient is placed upright in a chair so that the ptotic malar fat pad can be easily seen. The ideal shape and position of a youthful-appearing malar region is then marked directly on the patient's skin (**Fig. 10**). This triangular-shaped area may be treated with a topical lidocaine cream and then injected with a small amount of 1% Xylocaine with 1:100,000 epinephrine. Additionally, an infraorbital nerve block is performed by passing a 27-gauge needle into the canine fossa via the gingivobuccal sulcus and injecting a small volume of 1% Xylocaine. Although allowing for adequate anesthesia and vasoconstriction, the Radiesse is prepared by adding 0.2 mL of 2% Xylocaine with 1:100,000 units epinephrine to the 1.3-mL Radiesse syringe

and vigorously mixed. The addition of the lidocaine decreases the viscosity of the filler to allow for greater malleability and provides additional analgesia for molding across the inferior orbital rim. A single injection site in the middle of the area to be filled is selected. The needle is introduced adjacent to supraperiosteal tissues and the Radiesse mixture is slowly injected to create a "depot" of material that can then be molded into the desired shape. This technique is in contrast to the serial puncture or linear threading techniques commonly used in delivering fillers. Alternatively, the Radiesse can be injected transorally after an infraorbital nerve block and localization of the canine fossa (**Figs. 11, 12**). Care is taken not to inject too superficially within the dermis of the thin lower eyelid skin or too deeply into the postseptal orbital tissue. The authors do not advocate using Radiesse to treat the tear trough. Immediately following the procedure, the patient should apply ice and pressure to prevent bruising.

The significant advantage of the Xylocaine dilution is the ability to mold or sweep the product across the inferior orbital rim. An advanced technique would include a more limited depot medial

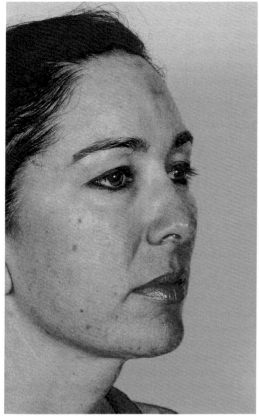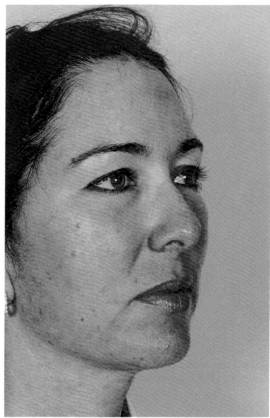

Fig. 8. Oblique photos of a patient demonstrating an isolated orbital groove before and after treatment with HA filler. After photo is 3 months postprocedure.

to the infraorbital nerve foramen onto maxillary periosteum with gentle sweeping of product upward. There should be great caution to avoid delivery of product proximal to the foramen because parasthesias have been a reported complication of injection adjacent to sensory nerves.

AUTOLOGOUS FAT TRANSFER TECHNIQUE

Autologous fat transfer is performed in the operating room under intravenous sedation supplemented with local anesthesia. Skin resurfacing and lower eyelid blepharoplasty are performed before fat transfer, if indicated. If an endoscopic brow-lift is planned, fat transfer is performed in all areas except the brow before the brow-lift and fat is placed in the forehead/brow region following the incisional lift. Any patient markings are performed in the holding area with the patient upright. The only recipient marks made are of the prejowl sulcus because the other areas are easily assessable with the patient supine while using preoperative photos. Donor areas are marked out in the holding area with the patient standing. The abdomen is the first choice of donor area, if available, followed by the medial and lateral thigh (**Fig. 13**).[11–14]

Once in the operating room and under sedation, the donor areas are infiltrated with 1% Xylocaine

Fig. 9. Radiesse setup for malar-inferior orbital rim augmentation.

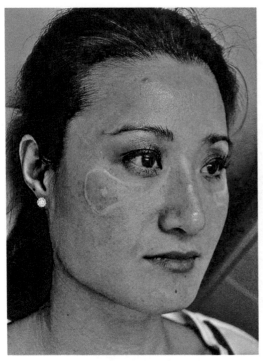

Fig. 10. Preprocedural markings, with transcutaneous entry site at malar prominence.

with 1:100,000 units of epinephrine mixed 1:1 with injectable 0.9% saline. The injection is performed with a 20-mL syringe and a 3-in by 25-gauge spinal needle. For the abdominal area, approximately 30 to 40 mL of solution is injected. Injection is placed in the immediate subcutaneous space and the prefascia space. No injection is placed in the midcutaneous plane where the fat is to be harvested to minimize possible toxicity to adipocytes from the Xylocaine. Usually, between 60 and 100 mL of fat is harvested. The leaner the patient, the less oil contained in the harvested fat. For heavier patients, the fat contains a higher degree of waste and larger quantities may be harvested.

Harvesting is performed with a small 15-blade stab-type entry point placed appropriately for the donor site. A bullet-tip 3-mm by 15-cm cannula (Tulip Medical Inc, San Diego, CA, USA) is used for harvesting with a 10-mL syringe. Gentle (2–3 cm) aspiration pressure is used to prevent lipolysis. The nondominant hand is used to stabilize the fat pad, while the dominant hand places the cannula in the midcutaneous plane. However, the fat should not be pinched up to prevent nonuniform harvesting and resultant contour irregularities. Before repositioning the cannula, 3 to 4 passes are made in one tract. When repositioning, the cannula must be brought nearly out of the

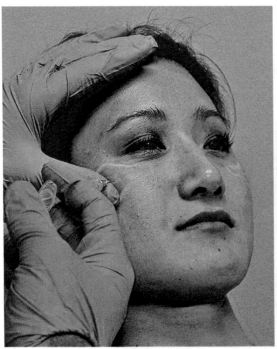
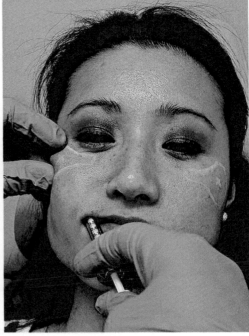

Fig. 11. Transcutaneous and transoral depot injection of Radiesse.

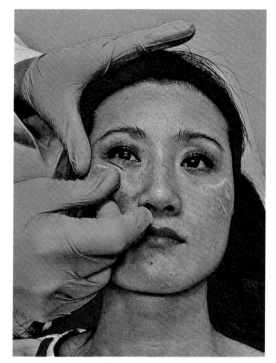

Fig. 12. Massage of Radiesse depot across inferior orbital rim.

incision to prevent the illusion of harvesting from a new area when the same local area is being used. This limits the amount of fat harvested and may lead to contour irregularities. One must be mindful of the cannula tip location at all times. Once completed, the entry incision is closed with a single subcuticular 5-0 monofilament polyglyconate suture.

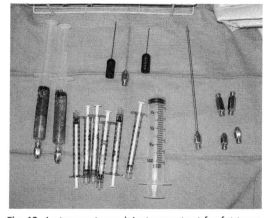

Fig. 13. Instruments used: Instrument set for fat transfer including harvesting cannula, injection cannulas, caps, and transfer hubs. (Tulip Medical Inc, San Diego, CA, USA; Byron Medical Inc, Tucson, AZ, USA).

The 10-mL syringes of fat are capped with a stainless steel plug intended for fat transfer, the plunger is removed, and the syringes placed in sterile sleeves in the centrifuge. The fat is spun at 3000 rpm for 2 to 3 minutes. The supernatant, which contains free fatty acid from lysed cells, is poured off into gauze. This should be performed before removing the plug to avoid loss of suction and the fat tumbling out. The plug is removed, the syringe placed in a sterile test tube rack, and the infranatant of blood and anesthetic solution is allowed to drain onto gauze (**Fig. 14**). The 10-mL syringes containing the purified fat are combined into a 60-mL syringe, and the air is removed by gentle stirring. Depending on the patient, approximately 50% to 75% of the harvested volume is injectable fat. The fat is transferred via a Luer-Lok transfer hub to 1-mL injection syringes. Three different injection cannulas are used for all injections: 1.2 mm by 6 cm and 0.9 mm by 4 cm spoon-tip cannulas (Tulip Medical Inc, San Diego, CA, USA) and Donofrio 16-gauge (Byron Medical Inc, Tucson, AZ, USA) straight blunt cannula.

Transfer is begun by infiltrating the entry sites with a small wheel of 1% Xylocaine with 1:100,000 units of epinephrine and performing nerve blocks of the supraorbital, infraorbital, and mental nerve foramen. Generally, fat is placed from entry points perpendicular to the desired area of placement. Transfer is begun in the inferior orbital rim area. An 18-gauge needle is used to make an entry site at the level of the nasal ala just lateral to the nasolabial crease. The orbital rim is approached from below, the nondominant hand is used to place a finger just inside the orbital rim, and the 1.2-mm cannula tip is "bounced" off the finger while dispensing small quantities of fat with multiple small passes in a plane immediately above the periosteum (**Fig. 15**). The medial orbital rim is treated, followed by the lateral rim. A second, more lateral entry site is often used to continue approaching the lateral rim from a perpendicular direction. In each location, medial and lateral, 1 mL of fat is placed. A third mL is then dispensed along the entire inferior orbital rim to even out and augment the area. Less fat is rarely used in this location and more may be added if needed. Often the 0.9-mm cannula is used to add fat into a slightly more superficial location to further augment the area. Quantities as large as 6 mL per side have been placed in this area, but more experience and care is indicated with these larger quantities because the risk of contour irregularities increases substantially.

The lateral canthal area is treated with an entry site in the crow's feet rhytids (**Fig. 16**). The 1.2-mm cannula is again used to infiltrate 1 to 2 mL

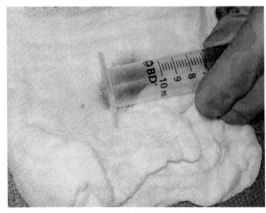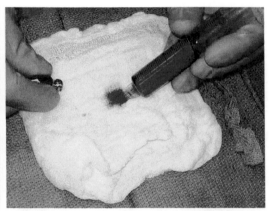

Fig. 14. The supernatant oil is drained off while the syringe is capped. The cap is then removed and the blood and fluid is drained from the infranatant.

of fat, blending it in with the inferior orbital rim fat. The superior orbital rim is then addressed by 1 or 2 entry sites in the forehead. The nondominant hand index finger is placed just inside the rim and the cannula is "bounced" off the finger while slowly placing fat in the plane just above the periosteum

if no brow-lift has been performed and in the deep subcutaneous space if the subperiosteal plane has been violated (**Fig. 17**). Usually, 2 mL is placed along the superior orbital rim. Fat may also be infiltrated in a superficial subcutaneous plane in the forehead and glabella, but this is an advanced technique and should be used after gaining experience. The temporal area is blended in with the other periorbital areas with 1 to 2 mL of fat and the 1.2-mm cannula.

The 16-gauge Coleman-Donofrio cannula is used to complete the transfer. This cannula is less fragile, and the remainder of the injections can be performed with greater ease and at a faster pace. The anterior cheek is addressed next by placing the nondominant index finger along the lateral aspect of the nasolabial fold. The cannula is inserted via the crow's feet entry site and 2 to 3 mL of fat is placed throughout the anterior cheek in superficial, mid, and deep cutaneous planes overlying the hollow of the malar septum. The

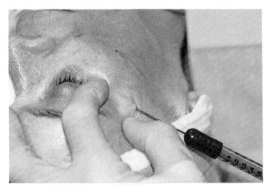

Fig. 16. The lateral canthus is approached from the crow's feet area. One to 2 mL is blended into the lateral inferior orbital rim injection and toward the superior orbital rim.

Fig. 15. The lower orbital rim is approached inferiorly using the Tulip 1.2 and 0.8 cannulas. The fat is injected in small parcels just above the periosteum with the nondominant index finger as a guide just inside the orbital rim.

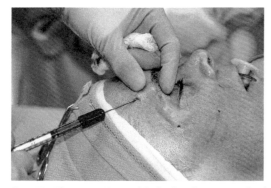

Fig. 17. The superior orbital rim is approached perpendicularly from the forehead. It is injected much like the inferior orbital rim with the nondominant hand just inside the rim, but smaller volumes are usually used.

lateral cheek is addressed by using the medial cheek entry site. The lateral extent of the anterior cheek augmentation is easily visualized. The lateral cheek is slowly built out from this point, injecting in multiple planes and tapering the malar eminence to a point over the zygomatic arch. This should create a teardrop appearance with the tapering superior aspect of the tear superior-lateral and a shadow under the lateral cheek that parallels the jaw line (**Fig. 18**). Usually, 2 to 3 mL is injected in this area. Larger volumes may be used for all these sites; the volumes given are conservative and generate substantial results with minimal risk. Further fat augmentation is performed in the buccal, perioral, and mandibular area but is beyond the scope of this article.

POSTOPERATIVE CARE

Postoperatively, the patient is asked to sleep with head upright and generously apply ice over the entire face. No wound care is necessary other than a small dab of ointment over the insertion sites. Patients experience a variable amount of bruising but a consistent amount of swelling. Patients are told to expect significant disfiguring swelling in the first week that decreases substantially by the end of the second week. Return to social activities can usually be achieved by the end of the second week in some patients and the third week in all. Some swelling and fat loss will occur through the sixth week and a small amount of volume will even be lost between 6 and 12 weeks. The volume stabilizes beyond this period, and long-term results can be expected with continued improvement in skin tone and texture even beyond 12 months, perhaps due to a stem-cell effect that is an area of on-going research. Autologous fat contains the highest proportion of stem cells in the body.[15] Some authors recommend freezing unused fat and re-injecting after 6 months. The authors have not found this necessary and rarely perform touch-up procedures. If a touch-up procedure is needed, fresh fat is harvested (**Fig. 19**A, B; **Fig. 20**A, B).

COMPLICATIONS OF FAT GRAFTING

Perhaps one of the major reasons many surgeons have been reluctant to adopt facial fat grafting as a surgical treatment option is the perceived transience of the result. Many surgeons have tried

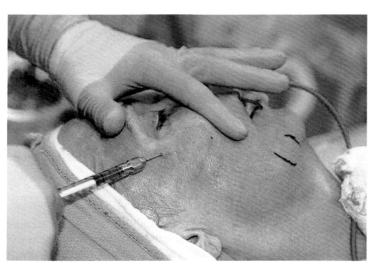
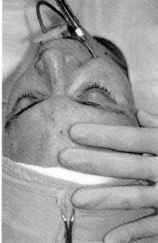

Fig. 18. The anterior cheek is approached from the crow's feet entry site. The nondominant index finger is laid against the bulge of the nasolabial fold and fat is injected in the deep subcutaneous and intramuscular plane all along this area. The lateral cheek is approached anteriorly, building on the lateral edge of the anterior cheek fat deposit to form a tapered tear drop.

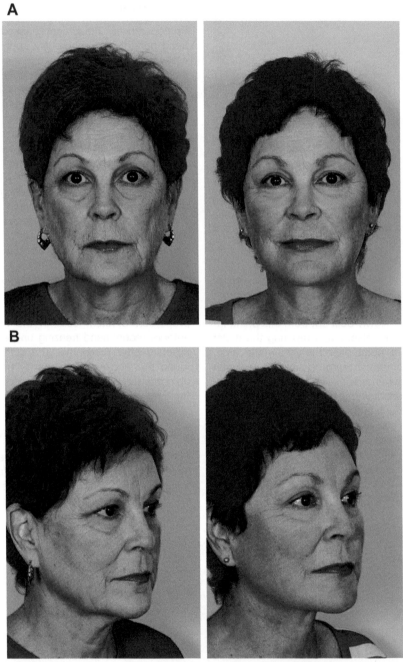

Fig. 19. Frontal and oblique views of 65-year-old woman 2 years after full-face fat transfer, full-face chemical peel, and lower facelift (*A, B*).

and given up on facial fat grafting because of failed attempts to achieve any durability. The authors believe that the reason for this failure, or perceived failure, stems from 2 problems: placing fat into facial areas that are not ideally treated with fat grafting, perioral area and lips, and poor operative technique.[16] Most complications in fat grafting can

be avoided by following the technique described, especially approaching the periorbital areas from perpendicular access points. Many types of potential complications can arise after fat transfer, including reported incidences of infection, nerve injury, and arterial embolism. Although extremely rare cases of embolism and nerve injury have

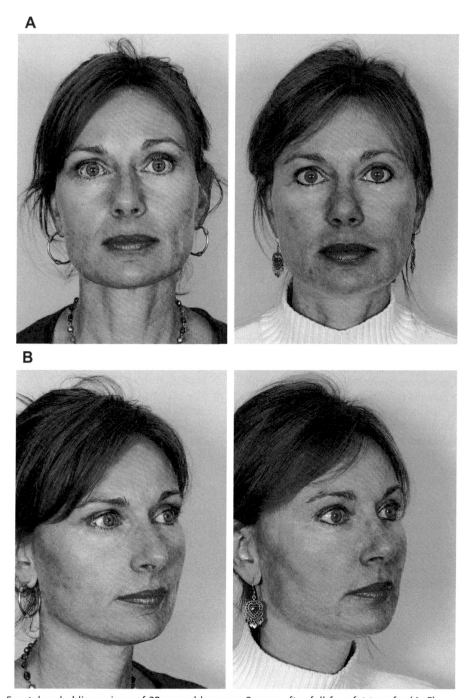

Fig. 20. Frontal and oblique views of 38-year-old woman 2 years after full-face fat transfer (*A, B*).

been reported, the authors believe that the chance of these occurring is further minimized when using blunt injection cannulas.[17] Although still rare, the more likely types of fat transfer complications are contour problems, particularly in the periorbital region. Complications can be divided into the following entities: lumps, bulges, persistent malar mound edema, overcorrection, and undercorrection.

A lump is defined as a small, discrete mass of injected fat that may occur as a result of too large a bolus or too superficial a location. Dilute steroid injection is a reasonable first step in treating these areas, but persistence may require direct surgical excision.

A bulge has a wider, cigar-roll appearance caused by imprecise placement of fat, overcorrection, or weight gain. Bulges caused by the first two may be treated by dilute steroid injection, direct excision, or microliposuction; the third is best managed with weight loss. Persistent swelling in the malar region should be distinguished from a bulge or overcorrection. The malar mound is a triangular-shaped elevation, anatomically delineated by the orbital septal-periosteal adhesion superiorly and the malar septum inferiorly. The most important step in avoiding this complication is to identify the presence of a malar mound preoperatively and determine whether the patient has a history of cyclical swelling. If present post-operatively, time may resolve the condition, but if it persists, dilute steroid injections at 4- to 6-week intervals may be useful. Overcorrection is best avoided through a conservative fat transfer, especially when beginning. If a patient feels they are overcorrected, a period of at least 6 months should be allowed, following which, if the conditions still persists, microliposuction of the area may be required. Undercorrection is the easiest problem to correct and should be anticipated in every patient. All patients are counseled on the likelihood that a second fat transfer procedure may be needed to obtain the ideal result, although this rarely happens.

SUMMARY

Volume loss is an important component of facial aging, especially in the periocular region. Careful analysis of each patient aids the surgeon in selecting and discussing appropriate volume augmentation procedures. Syringe-based fillers or autologous fat can be used with excellent results in well-suited patients with minimal complications.

REFERENCES

1. Ciuci PM, Obagi S. Rejuvenation of the periorbital complex with autologous fat transfer: current therapy. J Oral Maxillofac Surg 2008;66(8):1686–93.

2. Gunter JP, Antrobus SD. Aesthetic analysis of the eyebrows. Plast Reconstr Surg 1997;99(7):1808–16.

3. Matarasso SL, Carruthers JD, Jewell ML. Consensus recommendations for soft-tissue augmentation with nonanimal stabilized hyaluronic acid (Restylane). Plast Reconstr Surg 2006;117(Suppl 3):3S–34S.

4. Andre P. New trends in face rejuvenation by hyaluronic acid injections. J Cosmet Dermatol 2008;7(4):251–8.

5. Glavas IP. Filling agents. Ophthalmol Clin North Am 2005;18(2):249–57.

6. Fedok FG. Advances in minimally invasive facial rejuvenation. Curr Opin Otolaryngol Head Neck Surg 2008;16(4):359–68.

7. Lowe NJ, Grover R. Injectable Hyaluronic acid implant for malar and mental enhancement. Dermatol Surg 2006;32(7):881–5.

8. Verpaele A, Strand A. Restylane SubQ, a non-animal stabilized Hyaluronic acid gel for soft tissue augmentation of the mid- and lower face. Aesthet Surg J 2006;26(1S):S10–7.

9. Ridenour B, Kontis TC. Injectable calcium hydroxylapatite microspheres (Radiesse). Facial Plast Surg 2009;25(2):100–5.

10. Hevia OA. Retrospective review of calcium hydroxylapatite for correction of volume loss in the infraorbital region. Dermatol Surg 2009;35(10):1487–94.

11. Donofrio LM. Techniques in fat grafting. Aesthet Surg J 2008;28(6):681–4.

12. Coleman SR. Facial augmentation with structural fat grafting. Clin Plast Surg 2006;33(4):567–77.

13. Obagi S. Specific techniques for fat transfer. Facial Plast Surg Clin North Am 2008;16(4):401–7, v.

14. Lam SM, Glasgold MJ, Glasgold RA. Complementary fat grafting. Philadelphia (PA): Wolters Kluwer, Lippincott Willaims and Wilkins; 2007.

15. Coleman SR. Structural fat grafting: more than a permanent filler. Plast Reconstr Surg 2006;118(Suppl 3):108S–120S.

16. Coleman SR. Structural fat grafting. St. Louis (MO): Quality Medical Publishing, Inc; 2004.

17. Glasgold RA, Glasgold MJ, Lam SM. Complications following fat transfer. Oral Maxillofac Surg Clin North Am 2009;21(1):53–8, vi.

Periocular Rejuvenation: Lower Eyelid Blepharoplasty with Fat Repositioning and the Suborbicularis Oculi Fat

Jonathan R. Grant, MD[a],*, Keith A. LaFerriere, MD[b],*

KEYWORDS

- Lower eyelid blepharoplasty • SOOF
- Periocular rejuvenation • Fat repositioning
- Negative vector anatomy

Lower eyelid rejuvenation requires careful consideration of all layers of the eyelid and the transition to the midface. Hereditary anatomic variations in these structures and the changes typically observed with aging must be considered in optimizing periocular treatment outcomes. In the preoperative period, a thorough periocular examination is critical in determining optimal treatment strategies. The patient's medical history, expectations, and motivations must also be clearly defined before further surgical planning. Fat pseudoherniation, dermatochalasis, orbicularis hypertrophy, and prominent tear trough deformity are the most common indications for lower eyelid rejuvenation. Most commonly, fat pseudoherniation and prominence of the tear trough are addressed through lower eyelid blepharoplasties using either transcutaneous or transconjunctival techniques, with or without fat repositioning. Suborbicularis oculi fat (SOOF) lifting and fat transplantation have also been described as methods for softening the prominent tear trough in select cases. The indications and methods for each approach are described, with particular attention dedicated to the senior author's (KAL) technique for transconjunctival lower eyelid blepharoplasty with orbital fat repositioning, the most commonly indicated lower eyelid procedure in the author's experience. Adjunctive procedures for skin resurfacing and the utility of tear trough augmentation with fillers are also briefly described.

ANATOMIC CHANGES WITH AGING

The periorbital area demonstrates some of the earliest signs of facial aging. The integrity of the septum diminishes with advancing age such that orbital fat pseudoherniation leads to the appearance of bags or fullness in the lower eyelid. With advancing age, increased laxity in the structurally supportive tissues of the orbit also leads to relative settling of the globe, further exacerbating fat pseudoherniation through the areas of septal weakening.[1] Laxity in the lower eyelid septum can also be hereditary, as evidenced by the appearance of fat pseudoherniation in many adolescents and

a 2404 Station Circle, Dedham, MA 02026, USA
b Facial Plastic Surgery, St John's Clinic, 1965 South Fremont, Suite 120, Springfield, MO 65804, USA
* Corresponding author. 2404 Station Circle, Dedham, MA 02026 (J.R. Grant); Facial Plastic Surgery, St John's Clinic, 1965 South Fremont, Suite 120, Springfield, MO 65804 (K.A. LaFerriere).
E-mail addresses: jrgfish@gmail.com (J.R. Grant); Keith.LaFerriere@Mercy.net (K.A. LaFerriere)

Facial Plast Surg Clin N Am 18 (2010) 399–409
doi:10.1016/j.fsc.2010.04.006
1064-7406/10/$ – see front matter © 2010 Elsevier Inc. All rights reserved.

young adults. Orbital fat pseudoherniation contributes to the observed deepening of the nasojugal fold, or tear trough, that is associated with aging and gives the eyes a more fatigued, haggard appearance.[2]

Below the tear trough and orbital rim, the fatty tissues of the midface and cheek lose volume and descend as aging progresses. In a similar fashion, the SOOF loses volume and descends over time. In a youthful face, cadaveric studies have demonstrated that the SOOF attaches to the arcus marginalis at the level of the inferior orbital rim.[3] With aging, SOOF descent and volume loss contribute to deepening of the tear trough deformity and lengthening of the lower eyelid.[4] Concurrently, the orbicularis oculi muscle of the lower eyelid can hypertrophy, leading to heaviness, sagging, and deeper rhytids in the lower eyelid.[5] These changes in midfacial fat, SOOF, and orbicularis oculi contribute to the increasing potential for eyelid malposition, deepening of the tear trough, and rounding of the eye.[3] Lower eyelid skin also progressively loses its elasticity with aging, leading to progressive dermatochalasis with fine and deep rhytids.[5]

PREOPERATIVE EVALUATION
General Considerations

A complete discussion of all preoperative considerations for periocular rejuvenation procedures is beyond the scope of this article. Nevertheless, any history of dry eye symptoms, prior orbital or eye procedures, and comorbid conditions (ie Graves ophthalmopathy) or medications that can alter anticipated outcomes or wound healing should be investigated. Preoperative examination should address visual acuity, extraocular muscle function, tear film adequacy, lower eyelid tone, and lower eyelid resting position. Eyelid malposition or excessive laxity noted preoperatively should always be addressed before or concurrently with elective procedures.[5,6] A frank discussion regarding motivations, surgical risks, and anticipated benefits for proposed procedures must also take place between the surgeon and the patient, because inappropriate motivations, unrealistic expectations, and conditions that alter a patient's self-perception can preclude surgical candidacy.

Position of the Globe and the Inferior Orbital Rim

The relative positions of the globe and inferior orbital rim should always be assessed preoperatively, because their relationship is critical in determining the optimal procedures for treatment of the

aging lower eyelid and tear trough deformity. In the sagittal plane, if the anterior margin of the inferior orbital rim is posterior to the anterior-most point of the cornea, then the patient has a negative vector anatomy in the malar position relative to the anterior surface of the globe (**Fig. 1**).[2] Patients with a negative vector anatomy are more likely to have preoperative scleral show, because they usually have some degree of midfacial hypoplasia.[7] Preoperative scleral show should prompt evaluation of the position of the inferior orbital rim relative to the globe, because simple excision of the pseudoherniating lower eyelid fat in patients with negative vector anatomy often leads to exacerbation of the tear trough deformity and can lead to increased scleral show.[7] Given these anatomic considerations, patients with negative vector anatomy with fat pseudoherniation are excellent candidates for lower eyelid blepharoplasties with fat repositioning.

If the anterior margin of the globe has the same projection as the inferior orbital rim, the patient has neutral vector anatomy. In the senior author's experience, patients with neutral vector anatomy with fat pseudoherniation and tear trough deformities are also ideally suited for lower blepharoplasties with fat repositioning, because the repositioning minimizes the risk of future orbital hollowing and deepening of the tear trough deformity, seen with aggressive simple fat excision.

In contrast, patients seeking periocular rejuvenation with fat pseudoherniation and an inferior orbital rim positioned anterior to the anterior-most point of the cornea are not ideal candidates

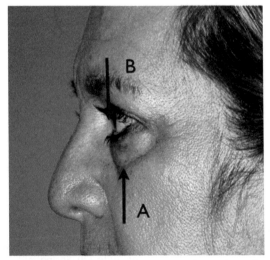

Fig. 1. Negative vector anatomy exists when the infraorbital rim (*A*) lies posterior to the anterior plane of the cornea (*B*).

for orbital fat repositioning. In such candidates with positive vector anatomy, conservative excision of fat is recommended when pseudoherniating fat is noted, because repositioning of orbital fat over the orbital rim may actually exaggerate, rather than improve, the already sunken appearance of the globe. In candidates with positive vector anatomy with tear trough deformity and little or no significant fat pseudoherniation, volume augmentation of the tear trough with fat transplantation, SOOF lifting, or filler augmentation is recommended.

Malar Bags

Focal areas of malar edema, or malar bags, should also be noted and discussed specifically with the patient in the preoperative setting. Malar bags can be a source of frustration for patients and surgeons. Surgical candidates should be advised that there is little consensus as to the most effective treatment for malar bags. The candidates should also be advised that sufficient improvement in lower eyelid fat pseudoherniation and dermatochalasis usually does not significantly alter the appearance of malar bags, even with extended skin or skin muscle flap techniques. In these patients, the surgeon should advise that the malar bags may actually become more noticeable once the lower eyelid concerns have been addressed (**Fig. 2**).

PROCEDURES
Lower Eyelid Blepharoplasty

Candidates for lower eyelid blepharoplasty should demonstrate lower eyelid fat pseudoherniation with or without orbicularis hypertrophy, excess lower eyelid skin, the appearance of circles under the eyes, or prominent depth in the tear trough deformity. Candidates presenting without

significant lower eyelid fat pseudoherniation and a prominent tear trough deformity require fat transplantation, filler augmentation, or SOOF lifting. Having the patient gaze upward exaggerates bulging in the lower eyelid secondary to fat pseudoherniation. Once the presence of significant fat pseudoherniation has been established, the surgeon must decide on whether to use transconjunctival or transcutaneous techniques and to recommend orbital fat excision or fat repositioning.

Transconjunctival techniques
With the exception of considerable dermatochalasis or orbicularis oculi hypertrophy, transconjunctival techniques work well for most lower eyelid blepharoplasty procedures. Transconjunctival approaches are associated with lower incidences of postoperative lower eyelid retraction and obviate any potential for external scar.[6,8] Especially in cases of preoperative scleral show, transconjunctival approaches are recommended, because the release of the lower eyelid retractors during this approach theoretically allows for elevation of the lower eyelid position relative to the globe.[8] Transconjunctival approaches are also ideally suited for young patients with familial development of lower lid fat pseudoherniation, because they rarely have significant dermatochalasis or orbicularis hypertrophy that requires surgical reduction. These patients are also excellent candidates for fat excision as opposed to fat repositioning. Although transcutaneous scars can be very inconspicuous, the risk of postoperative scar depigmentation (white scars) also leads many surgeons to recommend transconjunctival techniques in individuals with darker skin types (Fitzpatrick skin types V and VI).[7]

Transconjunctival approaches proceed in either the preseptal or retroseptal plane (**Fig. 3**). No

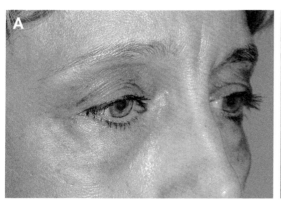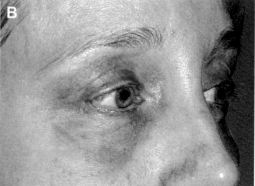

Fig. 2. Patient showing (*A*) preoperative and (*B*) postoperative persistence of malar bags after transconjunctival lower eyelid blepharoplasty with fat repositioning.

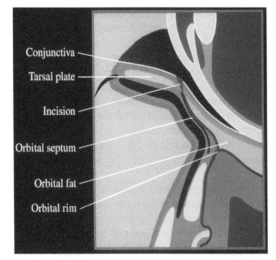

Fig. 3. Relevant anatomy for the transconjunctival approach to lower lid blepharoplasty, showing the option of preseptal or retroseptal exposure and subperiosteal or supraperiosteal options for fat repositioning or SOOF lifting. (*Courtesy of* M. Sean Freeman, MD, Charlotte, NC, USA.)

consensus as to the best technique was noted in the authors' literature review. Proponents of the preseptal method report that disruption of the or-bicularis–orbital septum fascial connections leads to further scar tissue formation on the septum, which bolsters against the pressures of fat pseudoherniation postoperatively.[8] Retroseptal method proponents argue that separating the orbital septum from the orbicularis in the preseptal method creates a cicatricial plane that can potentially result in inferior traction on the lid and postoperative lid malposition.[8,9] In the senior author's experience, eyelid malposition with either transconjunctival method is rare.

For either transconjunctival technique, the conjunctiva and lower eyelid tissues are first infiltrated with a local anesthetic (the upper malar face is also infiltrated at this point if fat repositioning is planned). Hyaluronidase may be mixed with the local anesthetic solution to facilitate dissipation of the anesthetic solution volume out of the soft tissues in the operative field. If the approach is preseptal, the conjunctival incision is made 2 to 3 mm below the inferior tarsal margin, spanning from just below the puncta to approximately 75% of the distance to the lateral canthus. The conjunctiva and lower lid retractors are then divided, usually with fine point electrocauterization, and a fine traction suture is placed through the retractors at the mid-pupil level and tacked superiorly to the drapes to protect the cornea and place the orbital septum on tension. With countertraction

on the septum in place, the dissection then proceeds inferiorly along the preseptal plane down to the orbital rim with blunt dissection using 2 cotton-tipped applicators, 1 for countertraction and the other to develop the plane. The orbital rim is then exposed far enough medially to expose the medial fat compartment and far enough laterally to expose the entire middle fat pad. Fat sculpting or repositioning is then performed through this exposure.

In the retroseptal transconjunctival approach, the conjunctival incision is approximately 5 mm below the tarsal plate, closer to the conjunctival fornix. Dissection then continues posterior to the septum on top of the orbital fat pads while reflecting the septum and orbicularis muscle anteriorly. Fat sculpting or excision can then be directly addressed. If fat transpositioning is to be done, a subperiosteal transposition pocket is made after incising through the arcus marginalis.

Transcutaneous techniques

Many surgeons still prefer transcutaneous techniques for various indications. Although skin pinch techniques with transconjunctival approaches are effective in removing limited amounts of redundant lower eyelid skin and orbicularis, more considerable dermatochalasis and orbicularis bulk with deeper skin furrows warrant a transcutaneous skin muscle flap or skin flap approach. Transcutaneous approach techniques for orbital fat repositioning have also been described.[5] When concurrent lid tightening procedures are planned, several surgeons also advocate the use of transconjunctival techniques rather than transconjunctival techniques, although lid tightening procedures have been described using transconjunctival techniques as well.[6,8] The critical factors in minimizing lower eyelid malposition in transcutaneous approaches are: maximizing sufficient intact pretarsal orbicularis, conservative trimming of redundant lower eyelid skin and hypertrophied orbicularis muscle, recognizing and correcting eyelid laxity, and suspending of the orbicularis muscle to the lateral orbital rim.[5,6]

When a skin muscle flap is used, the traction suture is placed through the pretarsal orbicularis to provide tension on the septum and protect the cornea. Otherwise, after the incision is made through the skin and orbicularis, dissection down to the orbital rim uses the same pushing technique with cotton-tipped applicators as described in transconjunctival techniques for exposure of the inferior orbital rim, arcus marginalis, and pseudo-herniating fat pads. A simple transcutaneous skin flap technique alone, without raising an orbicularis flap, can also be used in patients with significant skin excess without fat pseudoherniation for exposure of lower eyelid veins that are too large for laser or broadband light treatment. After raising the skin flap, the undesirable vessels can be accessed for direct removal or ablation (**Fig. 4**).

Fat Repositioning

Orbital fat repositioning can be done with either transcutaneous or transconjunctival lower eyelid blepharoplasty techniques and is an effective method of softening the depth of prominent tear troughs at the transition from lower eyelid to cheek. The fat repositioning technique was first described by Goldberg[7] in 2000. Variations on Goldberg's originally described technique for orbital fat transposition through a transconjunctival lower eyelid blepharoplasty have been reported.[2,5,8] Regardless of the initial approach, when the inferior orbital rim has been reached in the lower eyelid blepharoplasty dissection, the periosteum is incised at the orbital rim and a subperiosteal pocket is developed over the malar face inferiorly, approximately 1 to 2 cm below the orbital rim, ensuring that trauma to the infraorbital nerve is avoided. The arcus marginalis is then incised exposing the medial and middle fat compartments, taking care to avoid trauma to the inferior oblique muscle, and a pedicle is then developed for the pseudoherniating fat in the medial and middle orbital fat pad compartments. Regardless of whether the preseptal or retroseptal approach is used in transconjunctival blepharoplasty, the arcus marginalis must be released to mobilize orbital fat for transposition.[6] The mobilized pseudoherniating fat in the medial and middle compartments is then teased over the orbital rim and repositioned in the subperiosteal pocket.

The transposed fat can be either sutured directly to the undersurface of the orbicularis muscle, holding it in position over the orbital rim or secured in place with transcutaneous monofilament sutures. In the authors' experience, the preferred method is transcutaneous fixation, because this method seats the fat nicely over the orbital rim in a quick and secure fashion (**Fig. 5**). Typically, a first suture is used for repositioning of fat in the medial compartment, a second suture is used for the medial portion of the middle fat compartment just medial to the infraorbital nerve, and a third suture is used for the fat lateral to the infraorbital nerve in the middle compartment. These sutures are then typically secured in place without tension using flesh-colored Micropore tape (3M, St Paul, MN, USA) or tied over a small piece of rubber tubing, if simultaneous resurfacing is contemplated. The treatment of the resurfaced lower lid with ointment makes taping of these sutures inadequate. The temporal fat pad excess is excised, because repositioning is not feasible. Failure to recognize temporal fat excess mars an otherwise good result. The lower lid margin is then reevaluated to ensure that no limitation on lid mobility is noted with placement of the repositioning sutures.

In the authors' practice, fat repositioning is always used patients with in negative vector anatomy with fat pseudoherniation (**Fig. 6**) and almost always in patients with normal vector anatomy (**Figs. 7** and **8**). Positive vector anatomy is a contraindication to fat repositioning (**Fig. 9**).

As an alternative to repositioning in a subperiosteal pocket, fat repositioning within the SOOF layer has been described. However, even in small series, concerns have been raised regarding the potential for orbicularis denervation with this

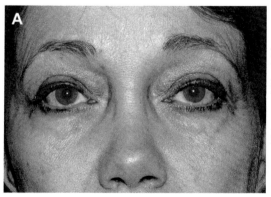
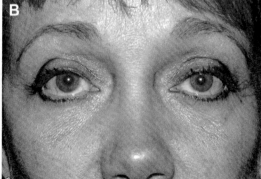

Fig. 4. Skin flap lower blepharoplasty with fat excision used for removal of prominent veins, noted in the left lower eyelid in the preoperative view (*A*). In the 1-year postoperative view (*B*), absence of the vein is noted, but mild increase in scleral show is evident.

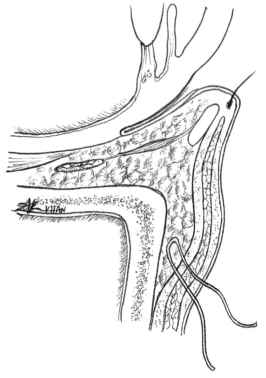

Fig. 5. Sagittal view of the lower periorbita demonstrating the subperiosteal fat repositioning held in place with transcutaneous sutures.

technique.[10] Subperiosteal repositioning of the fat avoids the lumpiness that can occur with placement above the periosteum.

Postoperatively, patients who undergo fat-repositioning should be advised to expect more swelling than is typical for lower eyelid blepharoplasty without fat repositioning, regardless of whether transcutaneous or transconjunctival techniques were used. However, this edema usually resolves rapidly after the fat repositioning sutures are removed on the fourth to the seventh postoperative day. Chemosis is not uncommon in the postoperative period and its resolution can usually be hastened with topical steroid ophthalmic drops given during a 3-day course. Lower eyelid mobility limitation can also be occasionally observed for up to 6 weeks following fat repositioning, but this limitation invariably resolves and its resolution can be hastened by massage and rarely by middle lamella injection with dilute triamcinolone preparations.

SOOF Lifting

Although the authors' experience with SOOF lifting is limited, the procedure, its indications, and its outcomes have been described in detail by Freeman.[3,11] In contrast to the ideal candidate for fat repositioning, the ideal candidate for SOOF lifting does not have an abundance of pseudoherniating orbital fat that could be used to fill the void of the prominent tear trough deformity.[3] Because the tear trough deformity is commonly associated with considerable pseudoherniating fat, fat repositioning is more universally practiced

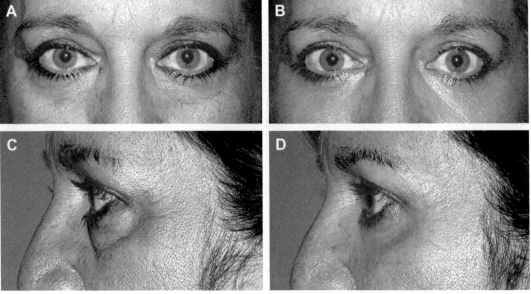

Fig. 6. Transconjunctival lower eyelid blepharoplasty with fat repositioning in a patient with negative vector anatomy. (*A, C*) Preoperative and (*B, D*) 1-year postoperative views.

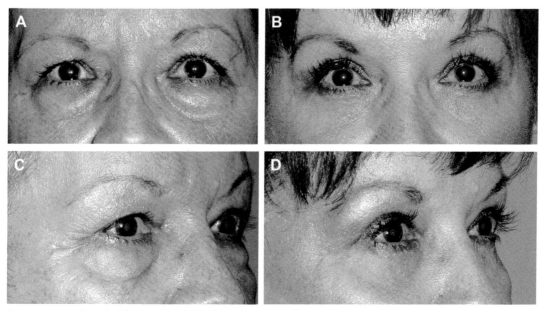

Fig. 7. Transconjunctival lower eyelid blepharoplasty with fat repositioning in a patient with neutral vector anatomy. (*A, C*) Preoperative and (*B, D*) 1-year postoperative views. Endoscopic forehead or brow lift and upper eyelid blepharoplasties were also performed.

than SOOF lifting. SOOF lifting can be performed in the presence of pseudoherniating fat but with some increased risk of diminished efficacy. According to Freeman,[11] younger patients with familial patterns of abundant pseudoherniating orbital fat are particularly difficult to treat effectively with SOOF lifting. Any excision of pseudoherniating fat in these patients at high risk should be very conservative to minimize treatment failure risk.

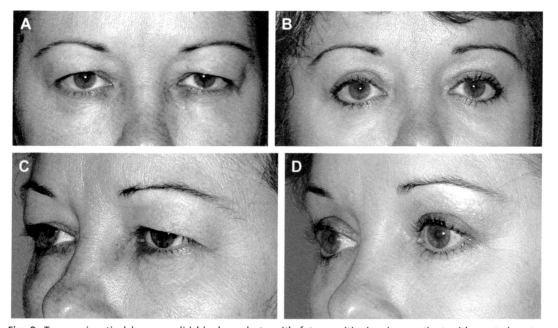

Fig. 8. Transconjunctival lower eyelid blepharoplasty with fat repositioning in a patient with neutral vector anatomy. (*A, C*) Preoperative and (*B, D*) 18-month postoperative views. Endoscopic forehead or brow lift, upper eyelid blepharoplasties, and ptosis repairs were also performed.

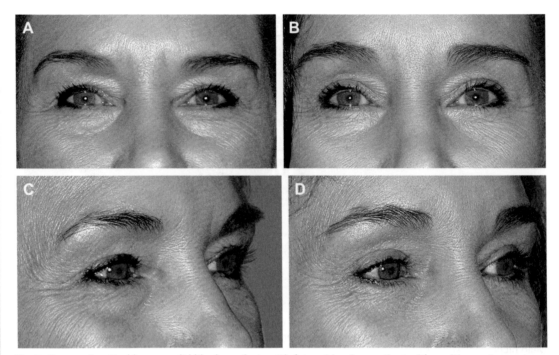

Fig. 9. Transconjunctival lower eyelid blepharoplasty with fat excision in a patient with positive vector anatomy. (*A, C*) Preoperative and (*B, D*) 1-year postoperative views. Endoscopic forehead or brow lift and upper eyelid blepharoplasties were also performed.

The descent and diminished volume of the malar fat pads and the SOOF exacerbates the tear trough deformity. SOOF lifting enables the surgeon to soften deep tear trough deformities by repositioning the SOOF superiorly. Although orbital fat repositioning allows for filling of the prominent tear trough with pseudoherniating orbital fat from above, SOOF lifting allows the surgeon to fill the tear trough with ptotic suborbicular fat from below (**Fig. 10**).

As described by Freeman, the initial incision is the same as for preseptal transconjunctival blepharoplasties. Dissection down to the inferior orbital rim is carried out in the preseptal plane. Then, rather than incising the arcus marginalis and developing a subperiosteal pocket, an incision is made just above the arcus marginalis down to, but not through, the periosteum along the medial half of the infraorbital rim. Dissection is then carried out in a blunt fashion with Q-tips on top

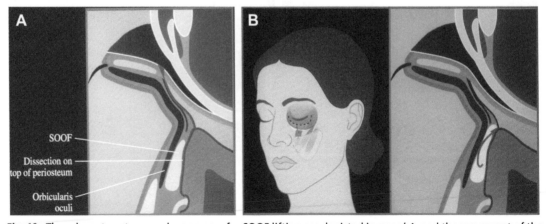

Fig. 10. The relevant anatomy and maneuvers for SOOF lifting are depicted in *panel A*, and the movement of the SOOF to fill the paucity of soft tissue at the infraorbital rim and nasal jugal groove is shown in *panel B*. (*Courtesy of* M. Sean Freeman, MD, Charlotte, NC, USA.)

of the periosteum past the inferior margin of the tear trough deformity. The ptotic SOOF is then identified, typically on the inside portion of the elevated flap adherent to the levator anguli oris. A 4-0 braided horizontal mattress suspension suture is then placed from the SOOF to the arcus marginalis of the infraorbital rim along the width of the tear trough deformity. The SOOF is then secured in place with the suspension suture such that it is raised to the level of the inferior orbital rim. In securing the SOOF suspension suture, care must be taken to avoid inadvertent tearing of the periosteum as the stitch is tied down. Once the SOOF suspension is secured, the conjunctival incision is closed with a single buried absorbable suture (**Fig. 11**).[3,11] Postoperatively, prolonged edema is expected for SOOF lifting as it is for fat repositioning procedures.

Fat Transplantation

Fat transplantation is ideally suited for instances of mild lower eyelid fat pseudoherniation with a tear trough deformity (**Fig. 12**). The depth of the tear trough deformity is caused by a paucity of soft tissue overlying the inferior orbital rim at the junction between the lower eyelid and cheek. Autologous fat can be injected up to the orbital rim to fill in the depth of the tear trough deformity and soften the transition from the lower eyelid to the cheek. Transplanted fat yields more-lasting volume enhancement than synthetic filler materials, because a large percentage of the injected autologous cells remain viable after injection. Hollowing in the tear trough and lower eyelid from overly aggressive fat excision in previous lower eyelid blepharoplasty procedures is also ideally suited for autologous fat transplantation.

A detailed discussion of the various preparation techniques for autologous fat transplantation is beyond the scope of this article. In brief, the autologous fat is typically harvested from the anterior abdomen or the medial or lateral thigh. After the harvested fat is centrifuged, the blood products and oily supernatant are separated from the fat cells for injection. The processed harvested fat cells are then injected in the periosteal plane along and below the orbital rim using multiple small volume injections, typically ejecting 0.03 mL of fat per pass, to give a uniform contour and distribution to the soft tissue augmentation. Because some degree of volume loss in the injected volume of fat usually occurs, a mild excess is typically injected. The upper cheek can be augmented simultaneously, because some degree of midfacial fat atrophy is typically present when the lower eyelid and tear trough hollows are the result of aging. In contrast to the effects of synthetic fillers, the effects of fat augmentation are permanent.

Adjunct Lower Eyelid Procedures

Skin pinch

The pinch technique is ideally suited and well established as an adjunct for treatment of redundant skin and limited orbicularis muscle in the setting of transconjunctival and SOOF lift lower eyelid blepharoplasties.[3,8] It is especially suited to surgical candidates at risk for pigmentary changes with laser or chemical peel resurfacing, such as patients with Fitzpatrick skin types IV to VI. When the transconjunctival portion of the procedure is complete, the pinch technique can be initialized. A local anesthetic solution containing a small volume of hyaluronidase is infiltrated into the subciliary skin in the pretarsal area. A horizontal fold of skin is then defined in the pretarsal area with a Brown-Adson forceps, approximately 1 to 2 mm below the lash line. The fold is then crushed with the forceps to delineate the redundant skin to be excised. Ideally, the fold should contain skin and little, if any, muscle to minimize the risk of postoperative eyelid malposition. The fold is excised with fine scissors, and the skin is

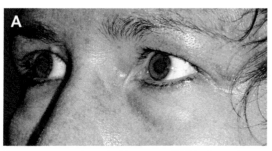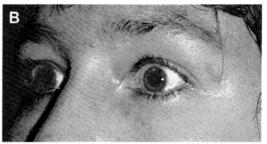

Fig. 11. Transconjunctival lower eyelid blepharoplasty with excision of pseudoherniated fat and SOOF lifting for correction of the tear trough deficiency. (*A*) Preoperative and (*B*) 1-year postoperative views. Forehead or brow lift and periorbital laser resurfacing were also performed. (*Courtesy of* M. Sean Freeman, MD, Charlotte, NC, USA.)

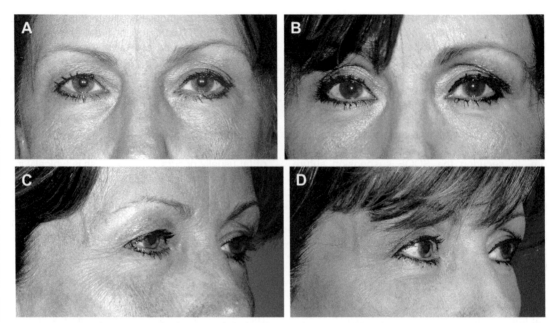

Fig. 12. Fat transplantation to the lower eyelids. (*A, C*) Preoperative and (*B, D*) 2-year postoperative views. Endoscopic forehead or brow lift and upper blepharoplasty were also performed.

closed with a fine permanent or absorbable suture in a running or interrupted fashion. As with all lid tightening procedures, undercorrection is preferable to overcorrection to minimize the risk of postoperative scleral show and complications related to lid retraction. In some cases of significant skin excess, simultaneous resurfacing can also be performed for the fine rhytids.

Skin resurfacing

Adjunctive skin resurfacing techniques such as resurfacing with erbium or CO_2 lasers or chemical peels are frequently used to augment lower eyelid skin tightening and treatment of fine rhytids in conjunction with transconjunctival lower blepharoplasties, with or without fat repositioning, or SOOF lifting. These procedures can be done concurrently with the primary lower eyelid procedures or as a secondary procedure at a later date for supplemental treatment of residual fine wrinkles and mild degrees of skin redundancy. As noted previously, there is a significant risk for pigment irregularities in patients with Fitzpatrick skin types IV through VI with skin resurfacing procedures; so patients with darker skin types may be more ideally suited for skin pinch excisions for persistent skin redundancy.[6,8,11]

Canthoplasty and lid tightening procedures

As previously noted, transconjunctival approaches for traditional and fat repositioning lower eyelid blepharoplasties, as well as SOOF lift blepharoplasties, minimize the risk of lid retraction

complications and frank ectropion. However, patients with preoperative eyelid malposition, lower eyelid tone and elasticity, or scleral show often benefit from concurrent lower eyelid tightening or shortening procedures such as lateral canthoplasty or other tarsal suspension procedures. Such procedures have been described in conjunction with transcutaneous and transconjunctival lower eyelid blepharoplasty approaches and should be compatible with SOOF lifting, because the approach is a transconjunctival approach.[5,8]

Synthetic injectable volume enhancement

Although an in-depth discussion of the various characteristics of different filler materials is beyond the scope of this article, a few salient points regarding treatment options for volume augmentation in the lower eyelid and upper cheek should be noted. Volume enhancement with injectable fillers is a widely accepted treatment option for tear trough deformity. Some surgical candidates may be more comfortable with fillers over other treatment options, because they perceive fillers as a less invasive, or nonsurgical, treatment option. Although results are not permanent, significant improvement in the prominent tear trough can be made with filler augmentation with variable durations of effect. The authors prefer hyaluronic acid derivates for volume enhancement of the tear trough deformity, because these preparations are more malleable and can be dissolved with hyaluronidase if the resultant injection effects are unsatisfactory. It is also the authors' observation that hyaluronic acid fillers last longer in the lower eyelid than in other areas of the face. Injectable fillers can also be used to restore volume in the SOOF and malar fat pads, effectively filling the soft tissue void over the inferior orbital rim from below, to soften the tear trough deformity and restore volume in midfacial fat compartments for a more youthful appearance.

SUMMARY

Lower eyelid rejuvenation requires careful consideration of relevant anatomy and the relationship to the upper cheek and inferior orbital rim. Transconjunctival lower eyelid blepharoplasty techniques are associated with lower risk of eyelid malposition; however, transcutaneous techniques are definitely indicated in certain circumstances. Several adjunct procedures have been described that are compatible with both techniques, especially for the treatment of dermatochalasis and lower eyelid laxity.

With transconjunctival and transcutaneous techniques, fat repositioning is also indicated when significant fat pseudoherniation and a prominent tear trough deformity are present in the setting of negative or neutral vector anatomy. In contrast, fat pseudoherniation in patients with positive vector anatomy should only be treated with direct excision or sculpting or should be camouflaged by treatment of the associated tear trough deformity with volume augmentation. In the authors' experience, prominent tear trough deformities without significant fat pseudoherniation are effectively treated with fat transplantation for permanent volume augmentation. Other injectable fillers yield favorable results as well but are not permanent. Although its indications are somewhat limited, SOOF lifting is another effective treatment option of the prominent tear trough

deformity, especially when there is little or no lower eyelid fat pseudoherniation present.[3,11]

REFERENCES

1. Doud Galli SK, Miller PJ. Blepharoplasty, transconjunctival approach. Updated 1/8/09. Available at: http://emedicine.medscape.com/article/838605. Accessed October 15, 2009.
2. LaFerriere KA, Kilpatrick JK. Transblepharoplasty: subperiosteal approach to rejuvenation of the aging midface. Facial Plast Surg 2003;19:157–70.
3. Freeman MS. Transconjunctival sub-orbicularis oculi fat (SOOF) pad lift blepharoplasty. Arch Facial Plast Surg 2000;2:16–21.
4. Rohrick RJ, Arbique GM, Wong C, et al. The anatomy of suborbicularis fat: implications for periorbital rejuvenation. Plast Reconstr Surg 2009;124(3): 946–51.
5. Perkins SW, Batniji RK. Rejuvenation of the lower eyelid complex. Facial Plast Surg 2005;21:279–85.
6. Jacono AA, Moskowitz B. Transconjunctival vs. transcutaneous approach in upper and lower blepharoplasty. Facial Plast Surg 2001;17:21–7.
7. Goldberg RA. Transconjunctival orbital fat repositioning: transposition of orbital fat pedicles into a subperiosteal pocket. Plast Reconstr Surg 2000; 105:743–8.
8. Fedok FG, Perkins SW. Transconjunctival blepharoplasty. Facial Plast Surg 1996;12:185–95.
9. Rousso DE, Fedok FG. Transconjunctival blepharoplasty: the method, indications, and complications. The Yearbook of the American Academy of Otolaryngology - Head and Neck Surgery 1993;900:195–211.
10. Mohadjer Y, Holds JB. Cosmetic lower eyelid blepharoplasty with fat repositioning via intra-SOOF dissection: surgical technique and initial outcomes. Ophthal Plast Reconstr Surg 2006;22: 409–13.
11. Freeman MS. Rejuvenation of the midface. Facial Plast Surg 2003;19:223–36.

Periocular Anatomy and Aging

Lily P. Love, MD[a],*, Edward H. Farrior, MD[b,c]

KEYWORDS
- Orbit anatomy • Eyelid anatomy • Periocular anatomy
- Aging eye

Eyelid anatomy is one of the more complex sets of anatomic relationships in the face. Differences are measured in millimeters, and structures are extremely fine and delicate (**Fig. 1**). The tissue can be very difficult to work with, requiring the utmost attention to detail. It is imperative to have an understanding of the complex anatomy and function of this region before any surgical or nonsurgical adventure is undertaken.

Anatomic descriptions involve western aesthetic tenets in Caucasians unless otherwise specified; although, as there are ever-increasing variations in aesthetic goals and many varying ethnicities, there is some generalization. The function of the lacrimal system and the orbital contents are beyond the scope of this article and are addressed only as they pertain to nonophthalmologic procedures.[1,2]

PERIORBITAL ANATOMY
Lid Topography

A few anatomic relationships are important when evaluating the orbital region. First, brow position may be evaluated. Common aesthetic relationships differ. In men, the brow is often most pleasing at the superior orbital rim in a less arched position. In women, the brow is ideally described as club-shaped, beginning in line with the alar creases medially at the orbital rim and arching above the rim with the apex over the lateral limbus and descending back down to the level of the orbital rim.[1,3,4]

The upper lid crease is formed by the insertion of the levator aponeurotic fibers into the skin (**Fig. 2**).

The crease is usually 8 to 9 mm in men and 9 to 12 mm in women. In the Asian population, the insertion is significantly closer to the lid margin, resulting in a lower or absent crease.[1] The lower lid fold may be 3 mm from the lid margin and is more common in the pediatric population (**Fig. 3**).[5]

The palpebral fissure is 28 to 30 mm wide and 9 to 10 mm high, with the lateral canthal angle 2 mm higher on a horizontal plane than the medial canthus (3 mm in the Asian population). The lateral canthal angle is 30° to 40°. The medial canthus lies about 15 mm from the midline (see **Fig. 3**).

The upper lid margin lies from the level of the superior limbus to 2 mm below normally.[6,7] Upper lid excursion may average 12 mm, whereas lower lid excursion is 5 mm.

Lid Anatomy

The eyelids are constructed with 3 anatomic and surgical layers: anterior, middle, and posterior lamellae (**Figs. 4** and **5**). The anterior lamella is composed of the skin, subcutaneous tissue, and orbicularis muscle. The skin is often less than 1 mm thick and may be thin enough to reveal underlying vessels and discoloration. Beneath the skin, there is some loose connective tissue in the preseptal and preorbital regions, which is absent in the pretarsal area. This subcutaneous tissue allows for the easy separation of the skin and muscle during surgical dissection.

The deepest layer of the anterior lamella is the orbicularis oculi muscle, which is divided into 3 regions (**Fig. 6**). The orbital portion overlaps with

[a] Otolaryngology, Facial Plastic and Reconstructive Surgery, Cedars Sinai Medical Group, Suite 640E, 18631 West 3rd Street, Los Angeles, CA 90048, USA
[b] Department of Otolaryngology, University of South Florida, 2908 West Azeele Street, Tampa, FL 33609-3110, USA
[c] Department of Otolaryngology, University of Virginia, VA, USA
* Corresponding author.
E-mail address: lilyplove@gmail.com

Facial Plast Surg Clin N Am 18 (2010) 411–417
doi:10.1016/j.fsc.2010.05.001
1064-7406/10/$ – see front matter © 2010 Elsevier Inc. All rights reserved.

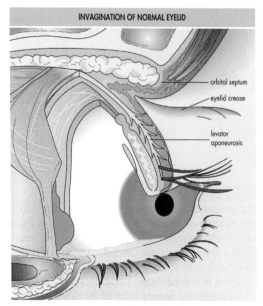

Fig. 1. Eyelid cross section and levator insertion. (*From* Yanoff M, Duker JS. Ophthalmology. 3rd edition. Mosby, an imprint of Elsevier; 2009. Copyright 2008; with permission.)

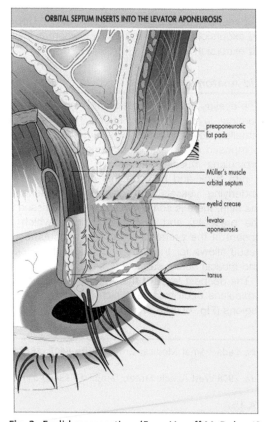

Fig. 2. Eyelid cross section. (*From* Yanoff M, Duker JS. Ophthalmology. 3rd edition. Mosby, an imprint of Elsevier; 2009. Copyright 2008; with permission.)

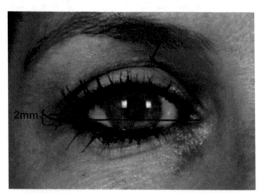

Fig. 3. Topographic anatomy of the lids with the lateral canthus positioned 2 mm above the medial canthus. Arrow demarks the position of the invagination of the lid crease.

other muscles of facial expression and may contribute to festoons of the lower lid in the aging process. The origin of this part of the muscle is the medial orbital margin and the medial palpebral ligament, with the insertion being lateral cheek skin.

The palpebral or preseptal portion is over the orbital septum, and the origin and insertion are the medial palpebral ligament and lateral palpebral raphe, respectively (see **Fig. 6**). The pretarsal region of the orbicularis muscle overlies the tarsal plate (**Fig. 7**). Beneath the orbicularis oculi muscle is the submuscular areolar tissue. Superiorly, this tissue may be followed to terminate at the retro-orbicularis oculi fat and inferiorly may be followed to the suborbicularis oculi fat.

The posterior lamella of the upper lid is more complex mostly because of the insertions of the levator aponeurosis (see **Fig. 2**). The deepest layer

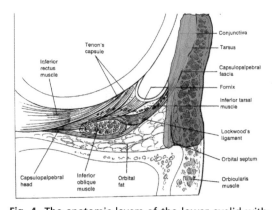

Fig. 4. The anatomic layers of the lower eyelid with the anterior lamella shaded red and the posterior layer shaded green. (*Adapted from* Cummings, C. Otolaryngology Head and Neck Surgery 4th edition. Philadelphia: Mosby, 2005; with permission.)

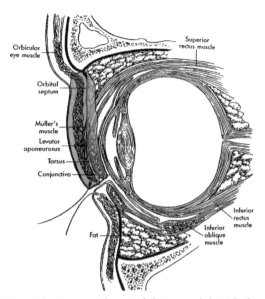

Fig. 5. The anatomic layers of the upper lid with the anterior lamella shaded red and the posterior lamella shaded green. (*Adapted from* Cummings, C. Otolaryngology Head and Neck Surgery 4th edition. Philadelphia: Mosby, 2005; with permission.)

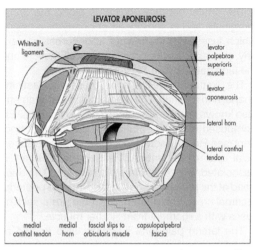

Fig. 7. Levator aponeurosis insertion. (*From* Yanoff M, Duker JS. Ophthalmology. 3rd edition. Mosby, an imprint of Elsevier; 2009. Copyright 2008; with permission.)

of the upper and lower lid posterior lamella is the conjunctiva. The conjunctiva is a thin epithelial mucosal membrane lining the inner lid and adheres to the tarsal plate. The tarsal plate is the area of dense fibrous tissue that gives the lid it's strength and rigidity. It is about 29 mm long and 1 mm thick. They attach to the medial and lateral palpebral ligaments (see **Fig. 7**).

The levator aponeurosis is the most superficial portion of the posterior lamella. It invests with the levator palpebrae superioris muscle, spreads laterally and medially, and attaches to the orbital septum forming the lid crease (see **Fig. 3**). Muller

muscle, which has sympathetic innervation, lies beneath the levator and is an upper lid retractor as well.[5,8]

The posterior lamella of the lower lid is similar to that of the upper lid with respect to the conjunctiva and tarsal plate. The conjunctiva is identical to that of the upper lid. The lower tarsal plate is shorter in height than the upper tarsal plate and is 3.5 to 5 mm high (see **Fig. 7; Fig. 8**).[5]

Lower lid retractors are a fascial extension from the capsulopalpebral fascia. There are some sympathetically innervated Muller muscles inferiorly as well.

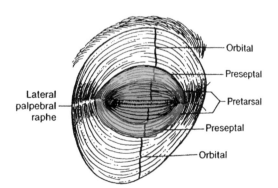

Fig. 6. The orbicularis oculi muscle and it's compartments. (*Adapted from* Cummings, C. Otolaryngology Head and Neck Surgery 4th edition. Philadelphia: Mosby, 2005; with permission.)

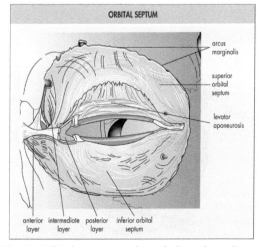

Fig. 8. Orbital septum and canthal tendons. (*From* Yanoff M, Duker JS. Ophthalmology. 3rd edition. Mosby, an imprint of Elsevier; 2009. Copyright 2008; with permission.)

The orbital septum originates along the arcus marginalis and is composed of connective tissue, which fuses with the levator aponeurosis superiorly. It is deep to the orbicularis oculi muscle and the lacrimal sac (see **Fig. 8**).

The ligaments in the orbit preserve elasticity, shape, and function. The medial palpebral ligament, also known as medial canthal tendon (see **Fig. 7**), is composed of a preseptal and a pretarsal component (see **Fig. 8**). Each of these is divided into superficial and deep limbs. The superficial head is associated with the pretarsal orbicularis. The deep head of the preseptal band inserts into the posterior lacrimal crest. The deep head of the pretarsal limb fuses with a ligament from Horner muscle.[5]

The lateral palpebral ligament, also known as the lateral canthal tendon, inserts 1.5 mm posterior to the lateral orbital rim (see **Fig. 7**). As with the medial ligament, the lateral ligament splits superiorly and inferiorly to fuse with the upper and lower tarsal plates.[5]

There are fat pads in the upper lid, posterior to the septum but anterior to the levator aponeurosis. Superiorly, there are medial and central fat pads, but no lateral fat pad because of the presence of the lacrimal gland.

Inferiorly, there are 3 fat pads: the medial, central, and lateral pads. The inferior oblique muscle divides the medial and central fat pads, and care must be taken during dissection (**Fig. 9**).[8–12]

Sensory innervations to the eyelids is provided by the terminal branches of the trigeminal nerve through the supraorbital and supratrochlear nerves (first division, V1) and infraorbital (second division, V2) (**Fig. 10**). The muscle innervation derives from

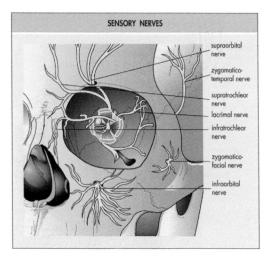

Fig. 10. Nerves of the orbit. (*From* Yanoff M, Duker JS. Ophthalmology. 3rd edition. Mosby, an imprint of Elsevier; 2009. Copyright 2008; with permission.)

the frontal and zygomatic branches of VII (**Fig. 11**). Muller muscle has postganglionic sympathetic innervation from the superior cervical chain.

The internal and external carotids provide blood supply to the eye. The internal carotid artery branches to the ophthalmic artery, which branches to the supraorbital, supratrochlear, and dorsal nasal branches and to the lacrimal artery. Superior and inferior marginal vessels also arise, which form the marginal arcades and run 4 mm and 2 mm from upper and lower lid margins, respectively. The external carotid artery branches into the facial artery, superficial temporal artery,

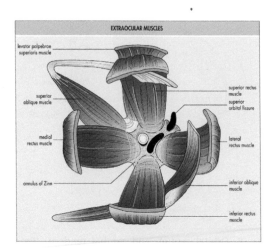

Fig. 9. Extraocular muscles. (*From* Yanoff M, Duker JS. Ophthalmology. 3rd edition. Mosby, an imprint of Elsevier; 2009. Copyright 2008; with permission.)

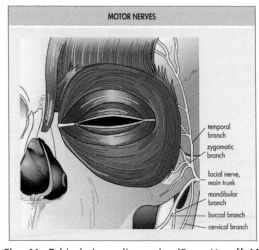

Fig. 11. Orbicularis oculi muscle. (*From* Yanoff M, Duker JS. Ophthalmology. 3rd edition. Mosby, an imprint of Elsevier; 2009. Copyright 2008; with permission.)

and infraorbital artery, which form an extensive anastomosis with the branches of the internal carotid artery (**Fig. 12**).[1]

The lymphatics of the upper lid and lateral half of the lower lid drain to the preauricular nodes, and the medial portion of the lower lid drains to the submandibular nodes.[5]

LACRIMAL SYSTEM

The lacrimal gland produces tears, which drain via lacrimal ducts in the upper portion of the lid. Tears moisten the globe and conjunctiva. The tears are then collected via the puncta of the upper and lower canaliculi at the medial aspect of the palpebral fissure. These canaliculi join to drain into the lacrimal sac, which sits in the bony lacrimal fossa. The drainage system continues down through the lacrimal duct, which finally drains inferior to the inferior turbinate of the nose.[13]

ORBITAL ANATOMY

There are 7 bones that contribute to the orbit (**Fig. 13**):

1. Orbital process of frontal bone
2. Lesser wing of sphenoid bone
3. Orbital plate and frontal process of the maxilla
4. Zygoma
5. Orbital plate of palatine bone
6. Lacrimal bone
7. Lamina papyracea of the ethmoid.

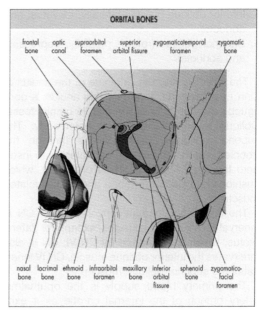

Fig. 13. Bony anatomy of the orbit. (*From* Yanoff M, Duker JS. Ophthalmology. 3rd edition. Mosby, an imprint of Elsevier; 2009. Copyright 2008; with permission.)

The orbit is typically approximately 40 mm in height, 35 mm in width, and 40 to 50 mm in depth. Interorbital distance is about 25 mm, and the total volume is about 30 cm³.

There are the superior orbital fissures containing cranial nerves (CNs) III, IV, and VI; the lacrimal nerve; frontal nerve; nasociliary nerve; orbital branch of middle meningeal artery; the recurrent branch of lacrimal artery; the superior orbital vein; and the superior ophthalmic vein. The inferior orbital fissure contains the infraorbital nerve, the zygomatic nerve, the parasympathetics to the lacrimal gland, the infraorbital artery, the infraorbital vein, and the inferior ophthalmic vein branch (see **Fig. 12**). The optic canal contains the optic nerve, the ophthalmic artery, and the central retinal vein.[5,8]

There are 6 extraocular muscles, which function to move the globe (see **Fig. 9**):

1. Medial rectus (adducts)
2. Lateral rectus (abducts)
3. Superior rectus (elevates, adducts, and rotates medially)
4. Inferior rectus (depresses, adducts, and rotates laterally)

A

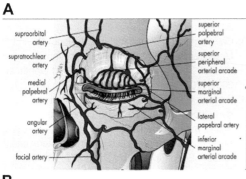

B

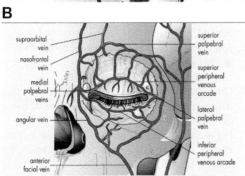

Fig. 12. (*A, B*) Vascularity. (*From* Yanoff M, Duker JS. Ophthalmology. 3rd edition. Mosby, an imprint of Elsevier; 2009. Copyright 2008; with permission.)

5. Inferior oblique (rotates laterally, elevates, and abducts)
6. Superior oblique (rotates medially, depresses, and abducts).

The 4 rectus muscles originate at the anulus of Zinn near the optic foramen; this anulus is contiguous with the dura of the middle cranial fossa. Oblique muscles originate independently. The superior oblique muscle passes through the trochlea and then travels posterolaterally to insert onto the eye.[5] There is diffuse orbital fat, which cushions and pads the globe and its associated muscles.[5]

The innervation primarily involves CNs. CN III innervates all rectus muscles except for lateral rectus, which is innervated by CN VI; CN III also innervates the inferior oblique muscle. CN IV innervates the superior oblique muscle.

The primary blood supply is the ophthalmic artery branch of the internal carotid as it exits the cavernous sinus. The ocular branches include the central retinal, ciliary, and collateral optic nerve branches. The orbital branches include the lacrimal artery, muscle arteries, and periosteal branches. The extraorbital branches include the anterior and posterior ethmoid arteries. Of importance when operating in the orbit is the location of the foramina through which the ethmoid arteries pass. "The distance from the orbital rim to the anterior ethmoid artery is approximately 20 to 25 mm. The distance between the anterior and posterior ethmoid arteries averages 12 mm, with a range of 8 to 19 mm. The optic ring averages 6 mm from the posterior ethmoid artery, with a range of 5 to 11 mm."[5]

AGING

Some of the first signs of aging in the late 20s and early 30s are usually around the eyes. The soft tissue changes are many.

Changes begin with the skin; there are notable increases in skin thinning and appearance of dynamic rhytids at the lateral canthi known as crow's feet. Increased laxity on the upper lid leads to hooding and occasionally pseudoptosis and is known as dermatochalasia. (This is different from blepharochalasis, which is not associated with aging but with a syndrome of recurrent painless edema and subsequent atrophy.) Lower lid skin laxity and laxity of the orbital septum can lead to the formation of bags. Bag formation may be caused by edema and skin stretching, known as malar bags,[8] or may involve the skin and ptotic orbicularis muscle, known as festoons.

Muscle laxity leads to some noticeable signs of aging. As mentioned earlier, orbicularis laxity in the lower lid contributes to festoons. Contraction of the orbicularis leads to changes in the overlying skin in the form of crow's feet.

Changes in fat position greatly contribute to signs of aging. With aging, there is a decrease in the amount of fat in the face, and there are changes in the surrounding area securing the fat. Laxity in the skin, muscle, or orbital septum may contribute to pseudoherniation or herniation, occasionally referred to as steatoblepharon. As the lower lid fat protrudes and the malar fat descends, the nasojugal groove becomes more prominent as well.[14]

Finally, there are important changes in the laxity of the connective tissue structures. Loosening of the septum, leading to bulging of fat was mentioned. Another important change is the increase in laxity of the canthal tendons. This increase may lead to a smaller appearance to the eye, scleral show, or even ectropion.[2,14]

REFERENCES

1. Asian blepharoplasty. Available at: http://emedicine. medscape.com/article/1282140-overview. Accessed June 15, 2009.
2. Erbagci I, Erbagci H, Kizilkan N, et al. The effect of age and gender on the anatomic structure of Caucasian healthy eyelids. Am J Ophthalmol 1994;117(2): 231–4.
3. Cartwright MJ, Kurumety UR, Nelson CC, et al. Measurements of upper eyelid and eyebrow dimensions in healthy white individuals. Eur J Ophthalmol 2007;17(2):143–50.
4. Beden U, Yalaz M, Güngör I, et al. Lateral canthal dynamics, correlation with periorbital anthropometric measurements, and effect of age and sleep preference side on eyelid metrics and lateral canthal tendon. Eur J Ophthalmol 2007;17(2):143–50.
5. Eyelid anatomy. Available at: http://emedicine. medscape.com/article/834932-overview. Accessed June 15, 2009.
6. Blepharoplasty; ptosis surgery work-up. Available at: http://emedicine.medscape.com/article/839075-diagnosis. Accessed June 15, 2009.
7. Orbit anatomy. Available at: http://emedicine. medscape.com/article/835021-overview. Accessed June 15, 2009.
8. Papel DIra, Larrabee Wayne, Holt G, et al. Facial plastic and reconstructive surgery. New York: Thieme Medical Publishers; 2002.
9. Dolan Robert. Facial plastic, reconstructive and trauma surgery. New York: Marcel Dekker; 2004.
10. Collin JRO. A manual of systematic eyelid surgery. Br J Ophthalmol 1999;83(3):347–52.

11. Van den Bosch WA, Leenders I, Mulder P. Topographic anatomy of the eyelids, and the effects of sex and age. Ophthal Plast Reconstr Surg 2005; 21(4):285–91.

12. Goldstein SM, Katowitz JA. The male eyebrow: a topographic anatomic analysis. Saudi Med J 2005;26(10):1535–8.

13. Bailey JByron. Head and neck surgery–otolaryngology. Philadelphia: Lippincott Williams & Wilkins; 2001.

14. Lambros V. Pathophysiology of aging [lecture]. Advances in Multi-Specialty Aesthetic and Reconstructive Plastic Surgery Symposium. Los Angeles (CA); September 13, 2009.

Management of the Asian Upper Eyelid

Amir M. Karam, MD[a],*, Samuel M. Lam, MD[b]

KEYWORDS

- Asian face • Asian eye cosmetic surgery
- Asian anatomy • Upper eyelid

Surgical management of the Asian upper eyelid requires a thorough understanding of two essential concepts:

1. Supratarsal crease creation
2. Evaluation and treatment of the aging upper eyelid complex.

Successful treatment mandates a unique set of strategies that include understanding the cultural aspects of the Asian patient, the anatomy of the Asian patient, and the techniques that would be appropriate based on these cultural and anatomic considerations.

An essential element to success in these cases is a firm understanding of the cultural bias and aesthetic standards of the Asian patient. Without this, it is common for the Western surgeon to become easily frustrated and potentially fail to meet the expectations of the patient. These issues are explored in depth in this article, and it is hoped the reader will thereby gain better insight and sensitivity.

CULTURAL ISSUES

Often, the Asian patient seeking cosmetic facial enhancement may have a separate layered agenda beyond simply desiring aesthetic improvement. Cultural and folkloric beliefs may not be overtly expressed but should be gently investigated to ensure patient satisfaction following a procedure. For example, the desire to obtain a larger nose through augmentation rhinoplasty may only be desired because of its association with greater wealth or the chance of obtaining it. Asian patients can be very obsessed with unblemished skin as a sign of beauty and also of good fortune.

Asians can also be much more secretive about undergoing plastic surgery than Caucasians, especially if the Asian has only recently immigrated to the West. Although HIPAA (Health Insurance Portability and Accountability Act) rules apply universally, the surgeon should be particularly circumspect when talking with any family member or friend regarding an Asian patient's surgery. Asian patients can also tend to be more negative in opinion of each other following cosmetic surgery, and the surgeon should prepare the patient for this possibility. Certain negative remarks by family members or social peers may be made to the patient consequent to the less socially acceptable nature of plastic surgery as compared with its more recently accepted position in the reality-television dominated Western culture.

Another important trend to consider is the desire and expectation to preserve ethnicity following cosmetic surgery. Despite the global images of Western beauty that permeate Asia, and the once widely held belief that facial cosmetic enhancement should "westernize" the core Asian facial characteristics, it is clear today that maintenance of Asian anatomic features are essential to a successful outcome. With respect to management of the Asian eyes, it is essential to keep in mind that eyelid creases that appear too high may not only be unacceptable to the

[a] Carmel Valley Facial Plastic Surgery, 4765 Carmel Mountain Road, Suite 201, San Diego, CA 92130, USA
[b] Willow Bend Wellness Center, Lam Facial Plastic Surgery Center & Hair Restoration Institute, 6101 Chapel Hill Boulevard, Suite 101, Plano, TX 75093, USA
* Corresponding author.
E-mail address: Md@drkaram.com

Facial Plast Surg Clin N Am 18 (2010) 419–426
doi:10.1016/j.fsc.2010.04.004
1064-7406/10/$ – see front matter © 2010 Elsevier Inc. All rights reserved.

Asian patient but also to the surgeon striving to achieve ethnically appropriate and natural-appearing results. With respect to the aging Asian eyelid, maintaining a natural eyelid crease following rejuvenative blepharoplasty lies at the core of this article and is discussed in the following sections.

Despite some of these cultural similarities among Asians, there are also very distinct differences that exist between nationalities. For example, the Vietnamese and Koreans are more predisposed toward having cosmetic enhancement. The Chinese are only now becoming enamored with cosmetic surgery, given their recent newfound wealth in a surging Chinese economy (and given its illegal status before 1979 in China). Even Asians who have emigrated from the Far East carry these cultural biases for or against plastic surgery from their native country. Second- or third-generation Asian Americans may begin to shake off some of these long-standing cultural biases as they assume more of a Western perception toward plastic surgery and toward life in general.

Delving into the underlying motivation for cosmetic surgery beyond merely improving one's aesthetic appearance can be a fundamental aspect to dealing with the Asian patient. Cultural biases may be overt or unspoken, but should be investigated as appropriate during cosmetic consultation with a prospective Asian patient.

SUPRATARSAL CREASE FORMATION

Asian upper eyelid blepharoplasty has a rich and varied history. The primary goal of this procedure is to create a supratarsal crease. The first reported case was performed and reported in the late nineteenth century.[1-7] Since then, several innovative surgeons began to describe their strategies, which can be broadly categorized into suture-based, full-incision, and partial-incision techniques. It should be noted that the presence of a supratarsal crease is a naturally occurring anatomic finding in the Asian population. The desire to have a "double eyelid" is largely cultural, as this feature is considered attractive.

The method advocated in this article is the full-incision technique. The rationale for this preference can be summarized by the following reasons:

1. Relative permanence compared with other methods
2. No need to rely on any buried permanent sutures to hold the fixation

3. Ease in identifying postseptal tissues through a wider aperture
4. Ability to modulate excessive skin (dermatochalasis) in the aging eyelid.

The major drawback of the full-incision method is the protracted recovery time during which the patient can look grossly abnormal for 1 to 2 weeks, and still not entirely natural for months if not a full year. Scarring has proven not to be an issue if the delicate tissue near the epicanthus is carefully avoided. Further, in the authors' opinion the incision line is more difficult to observe with the full-incision method than with the partial-incision method because there is no abrupt ending that is apparent with the more limited incision technique.

OPERATIVE TECHNIQUE

The first step is designing the proposed eyelid crease. There are several variations ranging from inside fold (the medial incision terminates lateral to the epicanthus) and outside fold (the medial incision extends medial to the epicanthus by 1 to 2 mm). There are 2 variations to the shape of the incision. The first is oval shape (slight flare of the crease height laterally above the ciliary margin), versus rounded in which the line runs parallel with the ciliary margin. The authors' preference is the inside fold paired with an oval configuration (**Fig. 1**).

Prior to marking, the patient should be placed in the supine position and the upper eyelid skin held relatively taut to the point that the eyelashes are just beginning to evert. To create a natural, low crease design (which constitutes the naturally occurring shape), the degree of skin excision to be performed should err on the side of conservatism, with about 3 mm (with the skin under stretch as mentioned above) between the

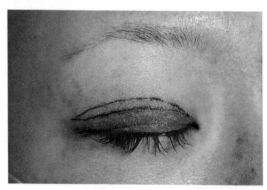

Fig. 1. The surgical marking of the inside fold paired with an oval configuration.

upper and lower limbs and with a distance of about 7 mm from the ciliary margin in most young adults.

Once the incisions have been carefully inspected for symmetry, the patient can undergo infiltration of local anesthesia. Deep sedation should be avoided as patient cooperation is vital to ensure symmetry toward the end of the procedure. A mixture of 0.5 mL of 1% lidocaine with 1:100,000 epinephrine and 0.5 mL of 0.25% bupivicaine with 1:100,000 epinephrine attached to a 30-gauge needle is used to infiltrate the upper eyelid skin by raising 2 to 3 subcutaneous wheals, which are then manually distributed by pinching the skin along the entire length of the incision (**Fig. 2**). This method, which avoids threading the needle, limits the chance of a hematoma that can lead to difficulty in gauging symmetry during the procedure. Of note, a total of only 1 mL of the aforementioned mixture of local anesthesia is infiltrated along each proposed incision to maintain symmetry.

After 10 minutes are allowed to transpire for proper hemostasis and anesthesia, a #15 blade is used to incise the skin down through the orbicularis oculi muscle, taking care not to pass the blade much further than that initial depth (**Fig. 3**).

Bipolar cautery is used coagulate the vascular arcades that run perpendicularly across the incision line in order to limit unnecessary bleeding and thereby mitigate swelling and distortion during this delicate procedure (**Fig. 4**). The depth of the incision can be further deepened with the #15 blade down toward the orbital septum before removing the skin island with curved Iris scissors. Additional cautery is used as needed. At this point, exactly the same procedure is performed on the contralateral side and is continued in this alternating fashion to ensure symmetry.

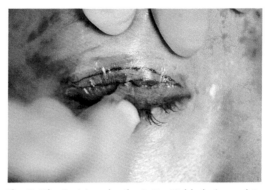

Fig. 3. The incision depth. A No.15 blade is used to incise the skin down through orbicularis oculi muscle.

The same Iris scissors are then used to excise an additional 1- to 2-mm strip of tissue along the inferior edge of the wound so as to remove any remaining orbicularis oculi fibers and some initial fibers of the underyling orbital septum (**Fig. 5**).

With the assistant gently balloting the eyeball above and below the incision line to help herniate the postseptal adipose through, the surgeon makes a small fenestration (**Fig. 6**) along the lateral extent of the wound edge just at the point where the strip of orbicularis was previously removed. With the countertraction and balloting of the eyeball mentioned above, the surgeon continues to excise thin films of tissue until the yellow postseptal adipose tissue is encountered. The reason for the small fenestration and the constant attention by the assistant to ballot around the incision to push the fat through the defect is that identifying the postseptal fat is the safety landmark to avoid injury to the deeper levator aponeurosis.

Once the fat is identified, a fine-toothed curved Mosquito clamp is inserted into the fenestration

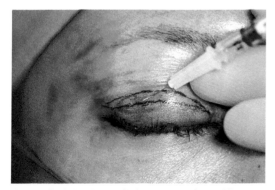

Fig. 2. The injection technique. Note that a 30-gauge needle is used to infiltrate the upper eyelid skin by raising 2 to 3 subcutaneous wheals, which are then manually distributed by pinching the skin along the entire length of the incision.

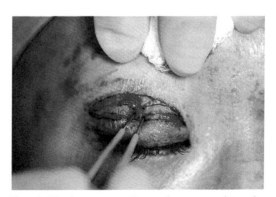

Fig. 4. Bipolar cautery is used to coagulate the vascular arcades that run perpendicularly across the incision line in order to limit unnecessary bleeding and thereby mitigate swelling and distortion during this delicate procedure.

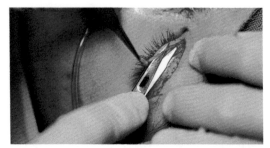

Fig. 5. The excision of a strip of orbicularis muscle along the inferior edge of the incision, thus exposing the underlying septum.

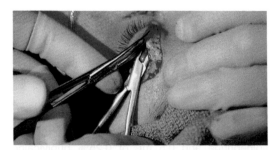

Fig. 7. A mosquito clamp is used to lift the septum up to protect the underlying levator aponeurosis. An iris scissor is used to divide the septum along the entire length of the incision.

and gently spread medially to lift the remaining orbital septum away from the deeper fat pad and levator aponeurosis (**Fig. 7**). Repeated entry and exit of the tines through the defect can help ensure that the correct tissue plane of dissection is maintained. With the tines open and the orbital septum tented upward, a bipolar cautery with Iris scissors can be used to open the remaining orbital septum to expose fully the deeper postseptal adipose and underlying levator aponeurosis.

A cotton-tipped applicator is used to sweep the preaponeurotic (postseptal) fat pad away from the glistening white levator (**Fig. 8**). At times a thin posterior leaf of the orbital septum can be seen between the levator and the fat pad. Gentle dissection using a fine-toothed Mosquito clamp followed by scissors of this thin orbital septum away from the fat pad can be undertaken to reveal the levator more fully. The same technique is undertaken on the contralateral side to this point.

Many surgeons believe that excessive adipose tissue must be removed to attain a more open eyelid configuration. However, in more than 80% of the cases simple levator-to-skin fixation is all that is necessary to attain the desired eyelid shape configuration and perceived opening of the palpebral aperture. Accordingly, preaponeurotic fat is rarely removed. This bias stems from seeing how much fat loss occurs with aging in the lateral

brow and upper eyelid, a condition treated with facial fat grafting in the aging eyelid. (If fat is removed, additional 2% plain lidocaine can be infiltrated directly into the fat pad to minimize discomfort, taking care not to permit any anesthetic to drip onto the levator.) At this point, the first levator-to-skin fixation suture can be placed. With the 5-0 nylon loaded backhanded on the needle driver, the patient is asked to open his or her eyes to determine the position of the midpupil on forward gaze so as to place the suture through the upper skin edge at the midpupil (**Fig. 9**). The suture bite is through the entire epidermis and dermis, as this suture will be removed 7 days postoperatively.

With the 5-0 nylon now loaded normally in a forehand fashion, a horizontal bite is placed through the levator at the approximate lower edge of exposed levator, again aligned at the midpupil. Next, with the 5-0 nylon loaded in a backhand fashion, the final throw of the needle is placed through the lower skin edge, again aligned with the midpupil. The patient is then asked to open his or her eyes after one suture knot to determine proper eyelash position. The eyelashes should be slightly everted, which should be the desired end

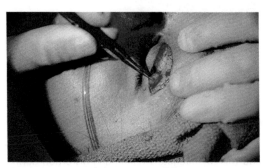

Fig. 6. Exposure of the postseptal fat.

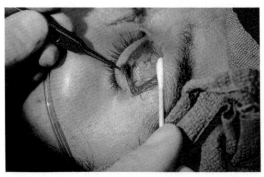

Fig. 8. The postseptal fat is swept away and the levator aponeurosis fully exposed.

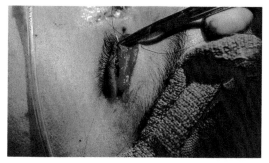

Fig. 9. Positioning of the 5-0 nylon suture used to create the new crease.

point. The crease height will appear grossly too high and should not be used as the desired end point (**Fig. 10**). If the eyelash position is deemed appropriate, the remaining 4 square knots are thrown to anchor the suture knot. The same technique is undertaken on the contralateral side, and symmetry of the creases is noted and can be adjusted as needed. A higher crease is created by placing the horizontal bite through the levator more superiorly, and lowered by placing the suture more inferiorly along the levator.

With the initial fixation suture placed bilaterally and symmetry observed, the 4 remaining fixation sutures per side can be placed in the same fashion. The second fixation suture is aligned with the medial limbus and the third fixation suture is positioned halfway between the lateral limbus and the lateral canthus. Two additional fixation sutures are used between these points to fine-tune any perceived asymmetry. A total of 5 fixation sutures are placed per side. The skin is then approximated with a running, nonlocking 7-0 nylon suture.

Fig. 11 shows a patient at 1 week, 6 weeks, and 6 months following the procedure.

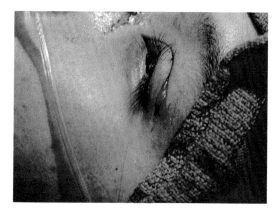

Fig. 10. Once each of the sutures are placed, the patient is asked to open the eyes to assess positioning and symmetry.

POSTOPERATIVE CARE

Postoperative care is straightforward, consisting of icing the eyelid areas for the first 48 to 72 hours, cleansing the incision line twice daily with hydrogen peroxide, and dressing it with bacitracin ointment for the first postoperative week. The patient returns on the seventh postoperative day to have all sutures removed, that is, the 5 fixation sutures per side (5-0 nylon) and the running skin closure (7-0 nylon). At times the patient may complain of difficulty opening his or her eyes due to excessive edema and/or temporary levator dysfunction, which can disappear over the first several days but can linger even up to 3 to 6 weeks following the procedure. The patient is reassured that it often takes a full year to achieve a natural crease configuration owing to persistent pretarsal edema that can linger for many months. Narrow, rectangular-shaped eyeglasses can camouflage some of the exorbitant edema in the immediate postoperative period; for female patients, mascara can be used to help hide the abnormal height of the crease during the initial few months following the surgery.

STRATEGIES FOR THE AGING ASIAN EYELID

As knowledge of the contribution of volume loss in the aging face increases, periorbital rejuvenation strategies that rely solely on reductive or excisional techniques (blepharoplasty or brow-lift surgery) is giving way to volume restoration and minimal surgical approaches (ie, skin only upper eyelid blepharoplasty). The premise behind this shift is to restore one's own youthful appearance without changing it. Evaluation of old photographs as a blueprint for rejuvenation has become increasingly necessary.

Often, brows that appear to have fallen and extra skin (dermatochalasis) that develops may in large part be due to volumetric loss of fat and soft tissue around the eyes. In the authors' view, traditional eyelid and brow surgery performed in isolation can alter a person's identity in a fundamental and irrevocable manner. It is noteworthy that most young women (not all) have a very low eyelid crease and relatively low brow position, but the shape and contour of that brow and eyelid are typically very full. Traditional brow and eyelid surgery, which is at heart reductive in nature, both serve to rejuvenate by cutting or lifting which, in turn, ultimately increase the distance between the ciliary margin and the supratarsal crease. This approach, by the very nature of the outcome, changes the patient's appearance if he or she did not have this lid configuration during youth. What

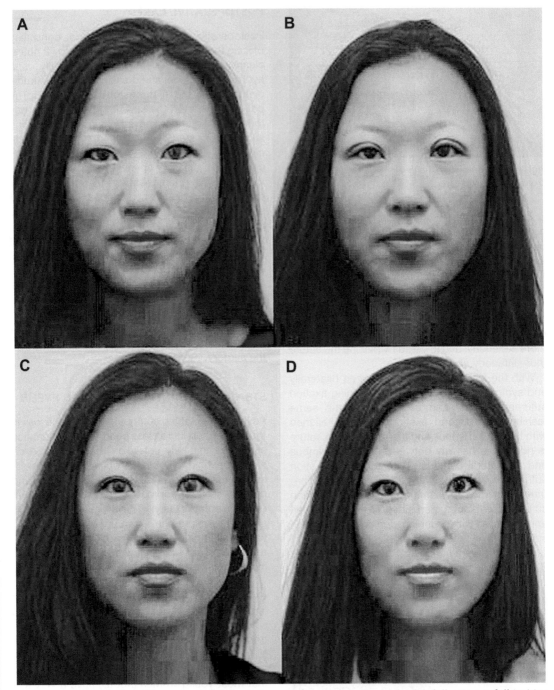

Fig. 11. A patient before (*A*), at 1 week (*B*), at 4 weeks (*C*), and at 6 months (*D*) following a full-incision procedure.

is interesting is that a high arched supratarsal crease *can* exist in the Caucasian race but generally is quite rare to find in the Asian race. Therefore, in the Caucasian patient the result of reductive periorbital surgery *can* still look natural, which is not the case for Asians or how Asians perceive their own face after cosmetic surgery. One of the most important attributes of the Asian eyelid is the relatively low crease structure that exists in almost all Asians of any age. The alternative to this shape would obviously be an Asian who does not possess an eyelid crease at all. It is the contention, then, that simply cutting away skin and performing a brow lift can adversely lift an eyelid crease in an Asian until it looks glaringly unnatural. Other considerations are also important. How does one manage an Asian without a natural crease who wants to have eyelid and brow rejuvenation? Or how does one manage an Asian patient who has already had previous eyelid crease formation? Is there a different strategy? This section elaborates a strategy that combines both cultural sensitivity and surgical judgment to treat an Asian patient for eyelid rejuvenation by classifying that individual into 1 of 3 categories: Asians with a natural eyelid crease, Asians without a crease, and Asians who have had an eyelid crease surgically fashioned in the past.

Asians with a Natural Crease

Although the surgical techniques are the same as in the Caucasian patient, the key to success is to maintain an eyelid crease in a low position. If the crease is lifted beyond 1 to 2 mm about the ciliary margin, it can render an Asian face unnatural in appearance. Maintaining eyelid crease position should be underscored as a fundamentally important objective with every endeavor. The way the authors maintain eyelid crease position is to avoid brow lifts in almost every case and to maintain or decrease eyelid position by using fat grafting in the upper eyelid and along the brow. Fat transfer to the upper eyelid/brow complex will actually reduce the height of the eyelid crease rather than raise the eyelid crease, as traditional blepharoplasty would do (**Fig. 12**). If the eyelid skin rests along the ciliary margin, it is recommended to remove a little bit of skin (but typically no fat) from the upper eyelid, usually about 2 to 3 mm in height of skin removal along with fat grafting, to reduce

and thereby maintain eyelid crease position. If the eyelid crease is 1 mm or greater above the ciliary margin, removal of skin is unnecessary (and counterproductive), and fat transfer alone is used. If the crease is much higher than 1 to 2 mm, additional fat can be used to lower the crease further. Traditionally 1 to 2 mm of fat is transferred to the brow and upper eyelid depending on the degree of brow and upper eyelid deflation as well as crease position. Looking at a patient's old photographs and discussing in detail with a patient his or her desired changes should frame each aesthetic consultation as it pertains to upper eyelid rejuvenation in the Asian patient.

Asians Without a Crease

The patient who does not have a natural crease can present a much more complicated scenario. In these cases, eyes look narrower so any brow and upper eyelid deflation can lead to further narrowing of the palpebral fissure. This appearance can be both aging and unaesthetic. Many surgeons simply decide an arbitrary height at which to remove skin without reference to thinking about the crease. This approach is problematic for 2 reasons:

1. Arbitrary removal of skin without crease fixation can leave behind a visible scar (even if placed right above the ciliary margin) because there is no crease to hide it.
2. The already narrow palpebral fissure will not be significantly altered by skin removal without attention to the postseptal fat.

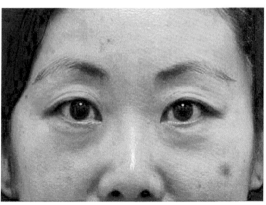 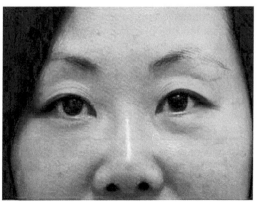

Before   After

Fig. 12. This Chinese patient demonstrates multiple incomplete, or partial, creases which, as the text states, should be treated as if she has no crease at all. In addition, she has a relatively negative vector eye shape. She was rejuvenated with only full facial fat transfer, and is shown *before* and *after* the procedure.

Instead, in the authors' opinion 2 options should be presented to the patient when it comes to treating the Asian patient without a defined crease.

One option is to create a crease. Making a crease opens up the eyelid shape enough to make an individual appear more awake or open-eyed. Using the full-incision method is ideal so that some dermatochalasis can be removed as needed. However, creating a crease requires that the surgeon knows how to perform this procedure well, which if not performed frequently can be technically difficult in achieving consistently superlative results. In addition, the patient must assent to wanting to change his or her "look" because the eyelid will perforce appear rounder in configuration. Finally, the long recovery time with a full-incision "double eyelid" procedure must be carefully elaborated, involving an artificial look that can persist even for several months and ultimately only look completely natural after one full year. This issue is particularly important to discuss with the male patient for 2 reasons. First, the Asian male patient looks completely unnatural with too high a crease (just like Caucasian male patients), and it takes some time for the crease to assume a natural height. Second, men have a more difficult time adjusting to a change in their appearance, especially after the adolescent years. This well-known psychological fact has been established in the rhinoplasty literature.

The second option, for patients who do not want a crease but still want eyelid rejuvenation, is fat grafting. Fat grafting to the upper eyelid and brow alone without skin removal can be the ideal way to improve the look without changing one's identity. Although the pretarsal tissue is already full in both youth and maturity in the Asian patient without a crease, converting an eyelid contour that is slightly concave in aging to more convex can bring back the look of a youthful eye. The patient must understand the limitations (if there are any) in simply adding fat to the brow and upper eyelid in the individual with an already narrow palpebral fissure born without a supratarsal crease.

Asians with Prior Surgery for Supratarsal Crease Formation

Asian patients who have a natural-appearing but surgically created crease that is not too high or over-resected can be easily treated as a patient who has a natural crease. Unfortunately, for many Asians today who are aging, their crease was surgically created during a time in which "westernization" procedures were in vogue, that is, when overzealous fat and skin removal were in fashion along with very high creases. These patients offer a uniquely difficult situation to address. Removing any more skin or lifting their brows can make their crease appear even more unnatural and should be avoided. It is interesting that 20 years following a westernization procedure, the eyelid crease height can approximate a "normal" or low position of about 1 or 2 mm with ongoing brow deflation. These individuals can be identified in that their crease appears to be of a normal, low height but there is something unmistakably unnatural about the appearance of their eyelids. The reason for this unnatural appearance is that the thick brow skin (all that remains after excessive eyelid skin removal) falls over the eyelid crease and the appearance of the crease appears too thick. Removing more skin or lifting the brow can literally unmask a bad prior result. If the surgeon is uncertain whether the crease is too high, he or she can simply lift up the brow skin to reveal how high the crease position is. For these Asian patients who have had a "westernized" eyelid, adding some fat along the brow and upper eyelid complex may be about the only course of action that can be the remaining "lesser of all evils." Even though the upper eyelid appears unnatural because it is thick, adding fat to the brow complex can actually make the appearance more natural in that it converts a thick concave structure (which is unnatural) to a thick, convex structure, which can actually partially camouflage the thick skin appearance.

REFERENCES

1. Lam SM. Mikamo's double-eyelid blepharoplasty & the westernization of Japan. Arch Facial Plast Surg 2002;4:201–2.
2. McCurdy JA Jr, Lam SM. Cosmetic surgery of the Asian face. 2nd edition. New York: Thieme Medical Publishers; 2005.
3. Lam SM, Glasgold MJ, Glasgold RA. Complementary fat grafting. Philadelphia: Lippincott, Williams, Wilkins; 2006.
4. Lam SM. Aesthetic facial surgery for the Asian male. Facial Plast Surg 2005;21:317–23.
5. Lam SM. Aesthetic strategies for the aging Asian face. Facial Plast Clin North Am 2007;15:283–91.
6. Shirakabe Y, Suzuki Y, Lam SM. A new paradigm for the aging Asian face. Aesthetic Plast Surg 2003;27:397–402.
7. Shu T, Lam SM. Liposuction and lipotransfer for facial rejuvenation in the Asian patient. Int J Cosmet Surg Aesthetic Dermatol 2003;5:165–73.

Rejuvenation of the Upper Eyelid

Sachin Parikh, MD, Sam P. Most, MD*

KEYWORDS

- Upper eyelid • Blepharoplasty • Eyelid rejuvenation

The eyes are the most captivating feature of the face. Furthermore, attractive eyes are an important feature of the youthful face. Although attention is drawn to the eyes, the surrounding structures that frame the eye are key contributors to facial beauty. The frame of the eye extends down to the lower eyelid-cheek junction and up to the upper eyelid–brow unit. Thus, the periocular region is a complex that should be broadly defined to include the eyebrow and midface. It is a surgeon's job to carefully analyze the underlying anatomy to determine the surgical approach to achieve the best aesthetic result.

The youthful upper eyelid is full, not hollow or overskeletonized. There is a crisp upper lid crease with elastic support of the underlying soft tissue, creating a smooth, taut pretarsal and preseptal upper eyelid. The eyebrow is often addressed in conjunction with the upper eyelid in upper face rejuvenation. This article focuses solely on surgical rejuvenation of the upper eyelid. The goal of rejuvenation of the upper eyelid should be a more youthful but natural-appearing result.

Upper eyelid surgery is the most requested and performed facial rejuvenation surgery in the United States.[1] The excision of the eyelids dates back 2000 years. The cauterization of excess eyelid skin to reduce drooping is described in the Sanskrit document, the *Sushruta*.[2] American surgeons began to write about cosmetic surgery in 1907, with Conrad Miller's *Cosmetic Surgery and the Correction of Feature Imperfections*.[3] Over the subsequent decades, surgeons advocated the removal of herniated fat pads and orbicularis oculi muscle excision. Over the past 20 years, the emphasis on technique has shifted to conservation of fat, skin and muscle excision

to avoid a deep, hollow, and skeletonized appearance to the eyelids.

EYELID ANATOMY

The position and form of the eyebrow has a deep impact on the appearance of the upper eyelid and eye below. A precise analysis of eyebrow position and form is a critical first step in the evaluation of the upper eyelids, a full analysis of which is beyond the scope of this article. A few salient points are discussed. The female brow is arched with the most superior aspect of the brow positioned directly above the lateral limbus. Laterally the brow sits above the orbital rim, and centrally there should be a high arch with a deep superior sulcus. The ideal position of the female brow differs from that of the male brow. The male brow is relatively straight, lying at the level of the orbital rim, and runs perpendicular to the nose with a minimal sulcus and a low subtle lid crease 8 mm above the lash line.[4]

Fig. 1 depicts many anatomic relationships that must be understood when evaluating the eyelid and assessing what needs to be addressed to restore youthfulness. The lateral canthus is typically 2 to 4 mm superior to the medial canthus. The adult palpebral fissure averages 10 to 12 mm vertically and 28 to 30 mm horizontally. The distance from the lateral canthus to the orbital rim is typically 5 mm. At rest, the upper eyelid covers the superior limbus by 1 to 2 mm. The highest point of the upper lid margin is just nasal to a vertical line drawn through the center of the pupil. This contour should be noted preoperatively when evaluating patients for rejuvenation of the upper eyelid so it can be addressed during surgery

Division of Facial Plastic and Reconstructive Surgery, Department of Otolaryngology/Head & Neck Surgery, Stanford University School of Medicine, 801 Welch Road, Stanford, CA 94305, USA
* Corresponding author.
E-mail address: smost@ohns.stanford.edu

Facial Plast Surg Clin N Am 18 (2010) 427–433
doi:10.1016/j.fsc.2010.04.005

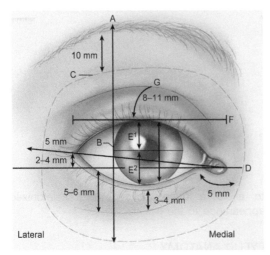

Fig. 1. Topography of the eyelid. (*A*) The highest point of the brow is at, or lateral to, the lateral limbus. (*B*) The inferior edge of the brow is typically 10 mm superior to the supraorbital rim. (*C*) Also shown are ranges for average palpebral height (10–12 mm), width (28–30 mm), (*D*) and upper lid fold (8–11 mm, with gender and racial differences). Note that the lateral canthus is 2 to 4 mm higher than the medial canthus. (*E*) Intrapalpebral distance measures 10 to 12 mm. E1, mean reflex distance 1; E2, mean reflex distance 2. (*F*) Palpebral width. (*G*) Upper lid fold is 8 to 11 mm. (*From* Most SP, Mobley SR, Larrabee WF Jr. Anatomy of the eyelids [review]. Facial Plast Surg Clin North Am 2005;13:487–92; Elsevier; with permission.)

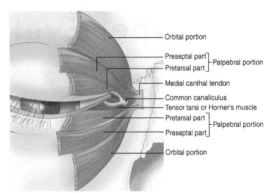

Fig. 2. Orbicularis oculi muscle. The muscle is traditionally divided into orbital and palpebral portions. The orbital portion arises from the anterior aspect of the medial canthal tendon and the periosteum above and below it. The palpebral portion is further subdivided into pretarsal and preseptal portions, each lying over the tarsal plate or orbital septum, respectively. (*From* Most SP, Mobley SR, Larrabee WF Jr. Anatomy of the eyelids. Facial Plast Surg Clin North Am 2005;13:487–92; Elsevier; with permission.)

to create a more aesthetic and appropriate lid position. The upper lid crease lies 8 to 11 mm above the lash line in whites but this varies with ethnic background. In Asians, the upper lid crease may be lower or absent owing to the lower insertion of the septum and variable or absent insertion of the levator aponeurosis into the upper lid skin.

The layers of the upper eyelid can be separated into an anterior lamella and a posterior lamella. The anterior lamella is comprised of the thinnest skin of the human body and the orbicularis oculi muscle. The posterior lamella is comprised of the levator aponeurosis, tarsus, Müller muscle, and conjuctiva.[5] Deep to the skin lies the orbicularis oculi muscle, which can be divided into an orbital portion and a palpebral portion. The palpebral portion is further subdivided into a pretarsal and preseptal portion lying over the tarsal plate and orbital septum, respectively (**Fig. 2**).

The postseptal fat of the superior orbit is divided into 2 compartments: the central (or preaponeurotic) and the medial (or nasal) fat pads separated by the trochlea and fascial strands from the Whitnall ligament.[4] During upper eyelid surgery,

surgeons must protect the trochlea to avoid superior oblique palsy or Brown syndrome.[6] The medial fat pad is paler and denser and recognition of these subtle differences is crucial for successful blepharoplasty with fat excision. The lacrimal gland occupies the lateral compartment. The retro-orbicularis oculi fat (ROOF) pad is a submuscular fat pad that sits deep to the interdigitation of the frontalis and orbicularis oculi muscles (**Fig. 3**).[4]

AGING OF THE EYES

The appearance of the upper eyelid may be affected by changes in the eyebrow position. Lateral ptosis of the eyebrow may add to fullness of the upper eyelid compounding the effect of the existing skin redundancy. In severe cases, this may cause visual field loss. The hallmarks of upper eyelid facial aging are lateral hooding, dermatochalasis, and fat pseudoherniation in the medial aspect of the upper eyelids. The upper eyelids become more redundant due to excess eyelid skin and eyebrow descent.[7] Rejuvenation of the upper eyelid is intended to elevate ptotic tissues and remove any tissue redundancy.

As a person ages, the loss of volume in the entire frontal region and loss of skin elasticity in the temporal region may account for brow ptosis, for those in whom this occurs. The tendency to counteract this by raising the eyebrows causes an accentuation of the hollowness under the eyes.[8] This also leads to a decrease in the lateral fullness of the upper eyelid. When the frontalis is relaxed,

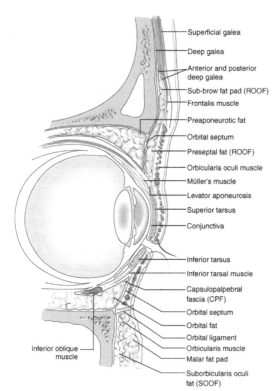

Superficial galea
Deep galea
Anterior and posterior deep galea
Sub-brow fat pad (ROOF)
Frontalis muscle
Preaponeurotic fat
Orbital septum
Preseptal fat (ROOF)
Orbicularis oculi muscle
Müller's muscle
Levator aponeurosis
Superior tarsus
Conjunctiva

Inferior tarsus
Inferior tarsal muscle
Capsulopalpebral fascia (CPF)
Orbital septum
Orbital fat
Orbital ligament
Orbicularis muscle
Malar fat pad
Suborbicularis oculi fat (SOOF)

Inferior oblique muscle

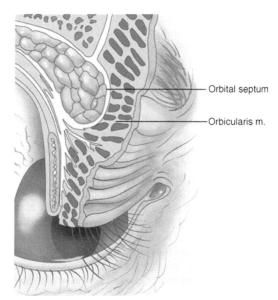

Orbital septum
Orbicularis m.

Fig. 4. The aging upper eyelid. Weakening of the orbital septum is thought to cause herniation of orbital fat in the upper and lower lids. (*From From* Most SP, Mobley SR, Larrabee WF Jr. Anatomy of the eyelids. Facial Plast Surg Clin North Am 2005;13:487–92; Elsevier; with permission.)

Fig. 3. Cross-sectional anatomy of the upper and lower lids. The capsulopalpebral fascia and inferior tarsal muscle are retractors of the lower lid whereas Müller muscle and the levator muscle and its aponeurosis are retractors of the upper lid. Note the preseptal positioning of the ROOF and suborbicularis oculi fat (SOOF). The orbitomalar ligament arises from the arcus marginalis of the inferior orbital rim and inserts on skin of the lower lid, forming the nasojugal fold. (*From* Most SP, Mobley SR, Larrabee WF Jr. Anatomy of the eyelids. Facial Plast Surg Clin North Am 2005;13:487–92; Elsevier; with permission.)

the redundant skin hangs lower, and the distance between the eyebrow and eyelashes is shortened. The weakening of the orbital septum also causes herniation of the orbital fat (**Fig. 4**). The lateral orbital region skin will develop rhytids, or crow's feet. The orbicularis oculi muscle may hypertrophy over time, causing the preseptal portion to become redundant and roll over the firmly attached pretarsal orbicularis, exacerbating the redundancy.[8] These factors all contribute to patients complaining of "looking tired, old, and not alert."

CLINICAL EVALUATION

As with any elective cosmetic procedure, the decision to perform a procedure to rejuvenate the upper eyelid is based on a thorough evaluation of the general medical history, ophthalmologic history, and psychological motivations of a patient. Medical history should include a history of chronic illnesses, hypertension, diabetes, bleeding disorders, and any anticoagulant medications. Key points in the history include any previous ophthalmologic procedures, history of thyroid eye disease, previous facial trauma, recent botulinm toxin type A treatments, and a history of dry eyes. Dry eye syndrome can be associated with medical systemic diseases, such as Sjögren syndrome, collagen vascular diseases, Wegener granulomatosis, and Stevens-Johnson syndrome. If a patient has dry eyes, a Schirmer test can be performed, but referral to an ophthalmologist is recommended.

An in-depth discussion between patient and surgeon must address their concerns and expectations. This allows both parties to ensure fluid communication, determine whether or not their assessments coincide, and reaffirm there are no unrealistic expectations. Surgeons must critically analyze and elicit patients' expectations and explain thoroughly that results can differ based on preoperative findings and ethnicity. For example, the Asian eyelid has more fullness of the upper eyelid, a lower lid crease, more narrow palpebral fissures, and possibly a medial epicanthal fold. Surgeons must discuss lid crease position with patients to determine their desires regarding postoperative lid crease position. Standardized preoperative photo documentation should be obtained. The authors also routinely obtain close-up views of the eyes in primary up gaze and down gaze in the frontal and in both lateral views.[9] Another helpful tool is reviewing patients' pictures from an earlier age. Analysis of such photos may help determine the contribution of brow ptosis to upper lid aging.

A physical examination must include a general overview of a patient's face, eyes, and eyelids. It is paramount to determine the brow contribution to aging of the upper lids when counseling patients for upper eyelid surgery, because this can alter a surgical plan. If there is any asymmetry of the palpebral fissures, it must be pointed out. Asymmetry is unmasked after a blepharoplasty and can become a source of dissatisfaction and a focus of attention for patients. It is imperative to also document visual acuity and extraocular movements and assess for dry eye, proptosis, and ptosis. If visual field obstruction is a concern, it is prudent to consult with an ophthalmologist for documentation and to determine whether or not the obstruction is clinically significant. The documentation of concurrent ptosis of the upper eyelid should also include measurements to the nearest 0.5 mm, if possible, using margin-to-reflex distance and levator excursion.[10] Surgeons must also check the conjuctiva for any erythema or edema. Finally, surgeons can assess how much can skin can be excised by using the pinch technique to grasp redundant skin with a forceps to ensure that there is no elevation of the lid margin. This reaffirms that excision of this skin can be safely undertaken without causing lagophthalmos.

SURGICAL TECHNIQUE

The authors prefer to obtain initial preoperative markings with patients in the upright position in neutral gaze. This is especially important if patients are to have a general anesthetic (eg, if the upper blepharoplasty is performed in conjunction with other procedures). In this position, the midpoint, medial extent, and lateral extent of the natural supratarsal creases on each side are marked. The lateral extent of the natural crease is noted— this approximates the lateral extent of the incision. The amount of lateral hooding is marked. The amount of redundant skin is noted. If a patient is to undergo browlift, the brows are elevated slightly and the amount of redundant skin noted. The brow is operated on first when done in conjunction with upper blepharoplasty because it reduces the amount of upper lid skin excision. If excess skin is removed from the upper eyelid without browlifting, the brow can be drawn further downward.

In the operating room, patients are placed supine. The lid crease markings are noted. Using a caliper, the previously performed markings are measured (**Fig. 5**). In occidental lids, the female upper lid crease is ideally placed 10 to 12 mm above the lid margin whereas in the male the ideal is 8 to 10 mm.[4] In many cases, the lid creases are noted as asymmetric. Typically, the authors select the side closest to the ideal for a patient and redraw the lower limb incision on the opposite side to match this.

Surgeons must be mindful of going far lateral past the lateral canthus because the incision becomes more visible in this area, especially in patients with thick skin. The lateral extent of the crease, noted preoperatively, is used as a guide. The pinch test is used to determine the amount of redundant skin that can be excised without causing lagophthalmos. In this test, a Green or Brown forceps is used to gently pinch the upper lid skin. The lower tine is placed on the proposed lower lid incision, and the upper tine position is varied until, when pinched, the upper lid lashes just begin to evert. This is the position of the superior incision. The medial extent of the incision is the punctum. If an excessive amount of skin is going to be excised medially, a W-plasty may need to be performed.[11] The point of maximal excision is lateral to the midpupillary line. The lateral extent of the incision can vary, depending on the extent of lateral hooding, patient acceptance of more visible scars, and the extent of the natural lid crease. Generally, it extends 5 to 10 mm beyond the lateral canthus. If the redundant skin extends well beyond the lateral canthus and the incision is performed more laterally, it may leave a visible scar. The thicker eyebrow skin that is removed laterally does not align favorably with the thinner eyelid skin inferiorly.

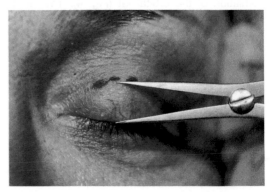

Fig. 5. A caliper is used to measure from the lid margin to the proposed upper lid crease.

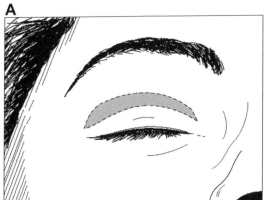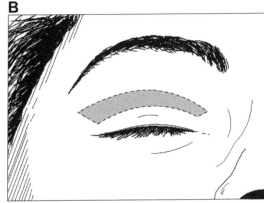

Fig. 6. Panels *A* & *B* represent two variations of the lenticular incision used in upper blepharoplasty. The medial extent is the punctum. The lower incision is 6 to 8 mm from the lid margin. The upper incision follows the contour of the brow.

The shape of the lower limb can vary medially and laterally (**Fig. 6**). Some surgeons prefer to converge the upper and lower limb incisions curvilinearly whereas others prefer a slight upturn to the lower limb medially and laterally. The authors prefer the latter, because it allows the upper and lower limb incision lengths to match more precisely, reducing the likelihood of redundancy of the upper limb skin at the medial and lateral extents of the incision (see **Fig. 6**).

Upper lid blepharoplasty can be performed under local anesthesia with or without sedation or under general anesthesia. A subcutaneous injection with 1% lidocaine with 1:100,000 units of epinephrine using a 1.25-inch, 27-gauge needle is performed. Local anesthetic should be injected superficial to the muscle to reduce the likelihood of formation of a hematoma. Incisions are made with a no.15 scalpel through the skin only. The strip of skin is removed with fine tip scissors (**Fig. 7**). In some cases, a 2- to 3-mm strip of orbicularis muscle is excised at the junction of the upper one-third and lower two-thirds of the wound site. The excision of orbicularis oculi muscle is intended to define a good eyelid crease definition. Patients with thin skin usually require little or no muscle excision, whereas patients with thick skin with redundant orbicularis muscle may require considerably more excision. In cases where medial fat excision is required, a small incision into the orbital septum is made medially. The medial fat is typically paler than the preaponeurotic fat and is more fibrous. Only fat that comes easily into the wound is excised. Meticulous hemostasis is maintained. The fat is labeled and kept so a surgeon can compare the amount of tissue removed from each eyelid. The authors avoid removal of the preaponeurotic fat to avoid a hollow, overoperated look. The skin incision may be closed with a running or interrupted suture using various absorbable or permanent sutures. The authors prefer a running 7-0 prolene suture. Immediately after surgery, antibiotic ophthalmic ointment is placed over the incisions and into the cornea. Patients are asked to apply antibiotic ointment twice per day. Sutures should be removed within 5 to 7 days. Patients may resume light aerobic activity at that time but must avoid bending over or lifting more than 8 pounds for 2 weeks. Nonsteroidal anti-inflammatory medicines must be avoided for 2 weeks pre- and postoperatively.

COMPLICATIONS

Complications from upper lid rejuvenation are infrequent and usually minor and transient. The most serious complication is partial or complete visual loss secondary to ischemic optic neuropathy or retrobulbar hemorrhage.[12] This complication is rare but treatment should be on an emergency

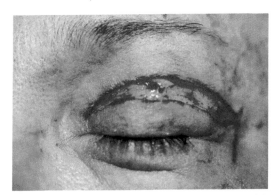

Fig. 7. A strip of skin is excised from the upper eyelid.

basis. These patients complain of severe orbital pain and visual deficits. Physical examination shows proptosis, tense globe, chemosis, increased intraocular pressures, and ophthalmoplegia. Emergency treatment involves exploration of the affected eye with evacuation of hematoma if present. If the vision is rapidly decompensating and intraocular pressures are high, lateral canthotomy and cantholysis with administration of ocular hypotensive agents may be necessary. The other visual complications can include an oculomotor disorder, epiphora, chemosis of lymphatic origin, and keratoconjuctivitis sicca.

A common complaint after surgery is a sensation of a dry or itchy eye. If this does not resolve after a few days, it should not be discounted as a corneal abrasion, but dry eye syndrome must be considered, which is a group of disorders caused by reduced tear production or excessive tear evaporation that may cause disease of the ocular surface. The pathophysiology can be explained by postoperative edema interfering with normal production and flow of tears. It is imperative to recognize preoperative risk factors through history and physical examination. Initially, dry eye syndrome is treated with artificial tears, ophthalmic lubricants, topical antibiotic, and steroid drops to help reduce the inflammatory response and prevent conjunctivitis.[13] Systemic corticosteroids can be added and tapered over 5 days. If the problem persists for more than 2 weeks, damage to the lacrimal gland should be ruled out. The presence of chemosis may alter management. If symptoms persist, an ophthalmologist should be consulted.

More common are eyelid issues from overresection or asymmetry.[12] These include ptosis of the upper lid, lagophthalmos, and eyelid fold anomalies. Ptosis is most often hidden on physical examination in patients with extreme dermatochalasis. If ptosis exists preoperatively, it can be addressed during the blepharoplasty. Lagophthalmos is frequent but transient and should be treated conservatively with lubricating substances and closure of the eyelids at night. Up to 3 to 4 mm of initial (eg, intraoperative and temporary) lagophthalmos may be observed after wound closure.[14] As the swelling resolves, the lagophthalmos improves. If there is a significant degree of lagophthalmos (up to 6 mm centrally and 1 to 2 mm medially), the excised eyelid skin should be replaced with a full-thickness skin graft.[14] If patients are refractory to medical treatment, reconstruction of the anterior lamella with a full-thickness skin graft should be considered.[12] If there is postoperative asymmetry, surgical revision can be discussed.

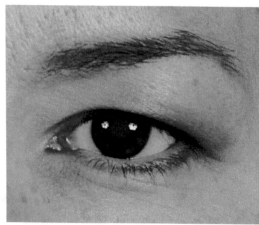
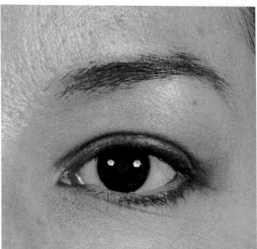

Fig. 8. Preoperative (*top*) and 4-month postoperative (*bottom*) images of patient who underwent conservative upper lid blepharoplasty and endoscopic browlift. Note that preoperatively, this patient had very full upper lids, particularly laterally. This fullness was not a result of aging, and reduction of this would not rejuvenate this patients eyelids. Preservation of epicanthal contour was important and this anatomy was maintained. Postoperatively, the patient has regained her more youthful, but full, upper eyelid/brow contour.

SUMMARY

Rejuvenation of the upper eyelid has undergone a change in philosophy over the past 20 years with the realization that preservation of facial volume, and periocular volume in particular, is desirable in most cases. An attractive face is characterized by lateral fullness of the upper eyelid/brow area with wide-open eyes and tight upper eyelid skin. The authors advocate minimal excision of skin, muscle, and fat to preserve a fuller, more natural look of the youthful eyelid (**Fig. 8**). Surgical rejuvenation of the upper eyelid can be achieved through various methods, including brow lift, frontotemporal lift, endoscopic forehead lift, Botox treatment, autologous fat tissue transplantation, and the use of injectable materials. The standard decision is whether or not to excise skin; skin and muscle; or skin, muscle, and fat.

There are a few new directions surgeons are taking in standard upper eyelid blepharoplasty that warrant mention. One group has espoused removal, cutting, and reimplantation of the medial fat pad within an imbricated layer of orbicularis oculi muscle.[15] This technique is designed to enhance a lateral, convex fullness and recreate key characteristics of the youthful eyelid. Fat can also be harvested and transplanted into upper eyelid tissue.[16] It remains to be seen if these techniques become widely adopted by facial plastic surgeons.

Rejuvenation of the upper eyelid is a dynamic surgical procedure that should be highly successful. A detailed understanding of the anatomic relationships of the eyelid is needed to achieve a nice aesthetic outcome. The keys to a good result are careful analysis on physical examination and of preoperative photos. The brow must also be analyzed and addressed if necessary. Standard resection of muscle and fat during upper lid blepharoplasty is no longer done routinely because the philosophy for conservative excision has become more accepted. The focus of resection should be on conservative reduction of redundant soft tissue. A youthful periocular region has subtle highlights and lateral fullness of the upper eyelid, creating an attractive frame for the eyes.

REFERENCES

1. American Academy of Facial Plastic and Reconstructive Surgery annual survey, 2004. Available at: www.aafprs.org. Accessed October 5, 2005.
2. Dupuis C, Rees TD. Historical notes on blepharoplasty. Plast Reconstr Surg 1971;47:246–51.
3. Miller CC. Cosmetic surgery and the correction of feature imperfections. 1907.
4. Most SP, Mobley SR, Larrabee WFJ. Anatomy of the eyelids. Facial Plast Surg Clin North Am 2005;13:487–92, v.
5. Becker DG, Kim S, Kallman JE. Aesthetic implications of surgical anatomy in blepharoplasty. Facial Plast Surg 1999;15:165–71.
6. Neely KA, Ernest JT, Mottier M. Combined superior oblique paresis and Brown's syndrome after blepharoplasty. Am J Ophthalmol 1990;109:347–9.
7. Lam SM, Chang EW, Rhee JS, et al. Perspective: rejuvenation of the periocular region: a unified approach to the eyebrow, midface, and eyelid complex. Ophthal Plast Reconstr Surg 2004;20:1–9.
8. Ross AT, Neal JG. Rejuvenation of the aging eyelid. Facial Plast Surg 2006;22:97–104.
9. Swamy RS, Most SP. Pre- and post-operative portrait photography: standardized photos for various procedures. Facial Plast Surg Clin North Am 2010;18(2).
10. Gentile RD. Upper lid blepharoplasty. Facial Plast Surg Clin North Am 2005;13:511–24, v–vi.
11. Rohrich RJ, Coberly DM, Fagien S, et al. Current concepts in aesthetic upper blepharoplasty. Plast Reconstr Surg 2004;113:32e–42e.
12. Morax S, Touitou V. Complications of blepharoplasty. Orbit 2006;25:303–18.
13. Hamawy AH, Farkas JP, Fagien S, et al. Preventing and managing dry eyes after periorbital surgery: a retrospective review. Plast Reconstr Surg 2009;123:353–9.
14. Romo T, Millman AL. Aesthetic facial plastic surgery: a multidisciplinary approach. 2000. p. 266–7. Available at: http://www.amazon.com/Aesthetic-Facial-Plastic-Surgery-Thomas/dp/product-description/0865778078. Accessed April 15, 2010.
15. Gulyas G. Improving the lateral fullness of the upper eyelid. Aesthetic Plast Surg 2006;30:641–8 [discussion: 649–50].
16. Trepsat F. Periorbital rejuvenation combining fat grafting and blepharoplasties. Aesthetic Plast Surg 2003;27:243–53.

Complications in Periocular Rejuvenation

William P. Mack, MD, PA*

KEYWORDS

- Blepharoplasty • Brow surgery • Lid retraction • Ptosis
- Orbital hemorrhage • Dry eye syndrome

The ultimate rejuvenation goal of cosmetic periocular surgery is to achieve an aesthetic balance between the forehead, periocular area, and midface. As patients who seek cosmetic surgery are focused on achieving their ultimate aesthetic result, it is imperative that cosmetic surgeons take the time to focus on the importance of educating patients regarding realistic outcomes and possible complications that may result from the planned procedure. This discussion should emphasize the aging changes that occur in the periocular region, including facial volume loss (deflation), volume shifting (descent), and skin, ligament, muscle, and bone changes, which lead to baggy lids, suborbicularis oculi fat descent, subcutaneous fat loss, and other age-related changes. Cosmetic surgeons should strive to restore fullness with avoidance of procedures/surgeries that result in hollowing and skeletonization. This goal can be achieved by efforts to reposition and reinforce, with an individualized surgical plan for each patient to achieve facial aesthetic balance with a youthful, refreshed appearance.

Because blepharoplasty ranks as one of the most popular cosmetic procedures in the United States, with more than 221,000 cases performed in 2008, thorough preoperative evaluation with meticulous surgical planning is imperative to decrease or even avoid the risk of potential complications (cosmetic and functional) that can occur with facial cosmetic surgery in the periocular region.[1] Possible functional issues following periocular surgery include keratopathy/dry eyes, infection, tearing/ocular irritation, lagophthalmos, hemorrhage/hematoma, diplopia, loss of vision, and/or blindness (**Box 1**).[2–8] Postoperative cosmetic problems include asymmetry, deep superior sulcus, periorbital hollowing, lateral canthal dystopia, and unnatural appearance. Complications with functional and cosmetic implications include eyelid malposition, retraction, and ptosis (**Box 2**). It is imperative that the cosmetic surgeon does not focus on the amount of tissue removed in periocular surgery; instead, the surgical goals should focus on the importance of preservation of tissue to retain a youthful symmetric fullness through repositioning and reinforcing to achieve optimal aesthetic results.

HISTORY

The importance of obtaining a thorough preoperative medical history should be emphasized because it is imperative to recognize patients who may be at an increased risk for complications from procedures to rejuvenate the periocular region. A history of systemic diseases, such as Graves disease, Sjögren syndrome, rheumatoid arthritis, rosacea, Bell palsy, and myasthenia gravis, or other neuromuscular diseases, should be ascertained. Patients should be questioned regarding a past history of ocular allergies, facial trauma, previous facial surgery (including skin cancer excision), or any previous periocular procedures.

Division of Oculoplastics Surgery, University of South Florida, Tampa, FL, USA
* South Tampa Medical Center, 508 South Habana Avenue Suite #170, Tampa, FL 33609.
E-mail address: drmack@tampabay.rr.com

Facial Plast Surg Clin N Am 18 (2010) 435–456
doi:10.1016/j.fsc.2010.05.002
1064-7406/10/$ – see front matter © 2010 Elsevier Inc. All rights reserved.

Box 1
Cosmetic complications

1. Asymmetry
2. Lower lid hollowing
3. Deep superior sulcus
4. Suture milia
5. Lid crease/fold asymmetry
6. Lateral canthal dystopia
7. Eyelid malposition
8. Medial canthal webbing
9. Scarring
10. Chemosis
11. Ptosis
12. Unnatural appearance

PERIOCULAR/OCULAR EXAMINATION

Following the complete review of their history, the prospective surgical candidate should have a complete periocular examination, including the brow, lid, and cheek regions as well as the ocular surface. During the initial consultation it is imperative to document and show any preoperative asymmetry. Patients for upper eyelid/brow rejuvenation surgery should undergo complete evaluation of the periocular area, including documenting the brow position and contour, as both contribute to a person's expression, whether angry, tired, sad, or happy. The diagnosis of underlying brow ptosis is crucial because patients may have evidence of frontalis muscle contraction to raise the brows secondary to underlying upper eyelid ptosis or significant dermatochalasis (**Fig. 1**). Because the distance between the brow and lid margin is increased from secondary brow compensation, an aged, tired appearance results. To unmask any underlying brow ptosis, apply manual pressure to the brow region and have the patient look in primary gaze (**Fig. 2**). In addition to the periocular evaluation, the prospective

Box 2
Functional complications

1. Dry eyes/keratopathy
2. Tearing/ocular irritation
3. Orbital hemorrhage/hematoma
4. Diplopia/strabismus
5. Visual loss/blindness
6. Lagophthalmos
7. Infection
8. Chemosis
9. Retraction
10. Ptosis
11. Eyelid malposition

patient should undergo a complete ocular examination with documentation of best corrected visual acuity, pupil examination, extraocular motility, and a slit lamp examination to evaluate the status of the cornea.

NORMAL EYELID ANATOMY

In the normal periocular region, the eyelid is shaped like an almond, with the highest point just nasal to the pupil and the brow position higher temporally (**Fig. 3**). The typical lid crease is around 8 mm, with at least 10 to 12 mm of skin superior to the eyelid crease to allow proper lid excursion and closure. The upper eyelid crease occurs where the uppermost fibers of the levator aponeurosis insert into the overlying lamellae and subcutaneous tissue. The lateral commissure is 1 to 2 mm higher than the medial commissure. The lower lid margin should be in apposition along the entire length of the eye.

To diagnose pathophysiology of eyelid malposition after lower eyelid blepharoplasty, the surgeon must be familiar with the surgical anatomy. The eyelid is divided into 3 layers: anterior, middle, and posterior lamella. The anterior lamella consists of the skin and orbicularis muscle, the middle lamella is the orbital septum, and the posterior lamella includes tarsus, conjunctiva, and the lower eyelid retractors. Lower eyelid retraction results from inflammation, scarring, shortening, and cicatricial tethering of the middle and posterior lamella (**Fig. 4**). Patients with a previous history of eyelid/facial surgery or facial trauma are at a higher risk for possible lid retraction. Anatomic factors that can contribute to an increased risk of lower eyelid retraction include prominent eyes, evidence of facial negative vector, midfacial hypoplasia, and scleral show.

BROW/UPPER EYELID EXAMINATION

In addition to the evaluation for brow ptosis or asymmetry, the examination for brow/upper eyelid surgery should include the eyelid crease and position, evidence of preexisting lagophthalmos (inability to completely close the eyes), floppy eyelid syndrome, deep superior sulcus, prolapsed lacrimal gland, and/or underlying eyelid ptosis (**Fig. 5**). The margin reflex distance (MRD1), which represents the distance from the light reflex of the patient's cornea to the center of the upper eyelid as the patient gazes in primary position, is used to assess the presence of upper eyelid ptosis. The normal MRD1 in an

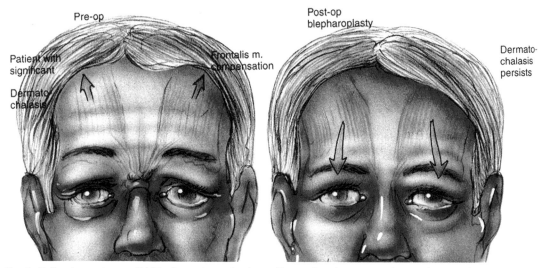

Fig. 1. Following upper eyelid blepharoplasty, the frontalis muscle relaxes secondary to decreased compensatory drive, therefore the eyebrow falls. The resulting droop of the eyebrow eats up much of the blepharoplasty results. (*From* Romo T, Millman AL. Aesthetic facial plastic surgery. 1st edition. New York: Thieme; 2000; with permission.)

adult is 1 to 2 mm below the superior corneal limbus in primary gaze (**Fig. 6**).

Assessment of the eyelid-brow complex should occur with the patient in a sitting position, with emphasis on the diagnosis of any brow ptosis, because this may give the false impression of lateral hooding of the upper lids. It is important to emphasize to patients who have evidence of brow ptosis and dermatochalasis that if they decline brow ptosis correction at the time of the blepharoplasty, the final aesthetic results may be compromised. In addition to examining for evidence of brow ptosis, it has been shown that the brow shape has a greater influence than absolute position on perceived expression.[9] It is also

important to note the distance from the brow to the upper lid margin because an increased distance, secondary to frontalis muscle compensation, is a characteristic sign of aging in the upper face. It is important to immobilize the brow position during the preoperative evaluation to negate the effects of frontalis muscle compensation, therefore exposing any underlying dermatochalsis or ptosis.

Any signs of ocular surface problems, dry eye syndrome, blepharitis, or eyelid inflammation should be documented in the upper eyelid evaluation. Attention should also be directed to noting any evidence of deep superior sulcus, as the degree of deepness of the superior sulcus is

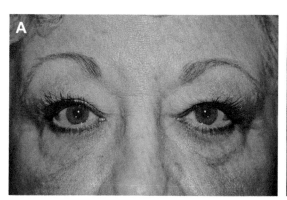
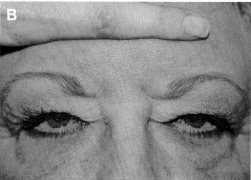

Fig. 2. (*A*) The diagnosis of underlying brow ptosis is crucial, because patients may have evidence of frontalis muscle contraction to raise the brows secondary to underlying upper eyelid ptosis or significant dermatochalasis. (*B*) To unmask any underlying brow ptosis, apply manual pressure to the brow region and have the patient look in primary gaze.

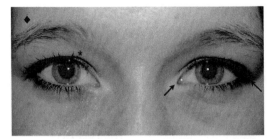

Fig. 3. Female patient showing characteristic almond-shaped eyelid anatomy, including normal MRD, lateral commissure 1 to 2 mm higher than medial commissure (*arrow*), the highest point of the upper eyelid just nasal to the pupil (*) and the brow position higher temporally (*diamond*).

determined by the interplay between the brow fat, preaponeurotic fat pads, orbital septum, and the levator aponeurosis. Many of the issues described earlier can be diagnosed and addressed before or during cosmetic brow or eyelid surgery.

LOWER EYELID/CHEEK EXAMINATION

With aging, the lower eyelid cheek junction develops an uneven contour secondary to descent of the cheek, with increased prominence of the lower lid fat, resulting in a nasojugal groove with a tear trough deformity. In addition to the evaluation for dry eye syndrome, patients seeking cosmetic lower eyelid surgery should be evaluated for evidence of eyelid malposition, descent of the

malar fat pads, poor maxillary bony support with a negative facial vector, stretching of the lateral canthal tendons, eyelid retraction, lagophthalmos, lower lid hollowing, alteration in the tear film/blink reflex, ineffectiveness of the tearing-lacrimal pump, evidence of corneal exposure, eyelid or punctal ectropion, scleral show, and lid laxity. Hester and colleagues[10] found that patients with enophthalmic orbits and significant horizontal lower lid laxity were at an increased risk for postoperative lower lid malposition (**Box 3**).

The distraction test is performed by pulling the eyelid anteriorly; if the distracted distance is greater than 6 to 8 mm, then lower lid laxity is evident (**Fig. 7**). The snap back test, which assesses the function of the orbicularis muscle and the amount of lid tone, is performed as the lower lid is pulled toward the inferior orbital rim and released. A fast snap of the lower eyelid to the proper position indicates normal tension, whereas poor snap back shows evidence of poor lid tone (**Fig. 8**). To examine for lagophthalmos, the patient is instructed to passively close the eyelids as if they were sleeping (**Fig. 9**).

It is also recommended to check the Bell phenomenon and the amount of lateral canthal tendon laxity. Defined as inferior malposition of the lower eyelid margin without eyelid eversion, lower eyelid retraction is assessed by placing upward traction on the lower eyelid. In normal conditions, the lower eyelid can be raised to at least the midpupil level. If this level is not achieved

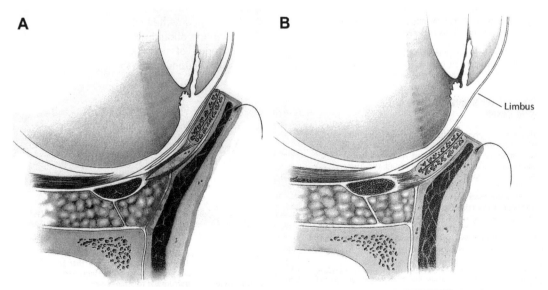

Fig. 4. (*A*) Normal lower eyelid with red highlighted area where cicatricial changes occur that result in lower lid retraction. (*B*) Lower lid retraction, which develops from postsurgical manipulation, is characterized by inflammation, scarring, shortening, and cicatricial tethering of the middle and posterior lamella. (*Courtesy of* Robert Goldberg, MD.)

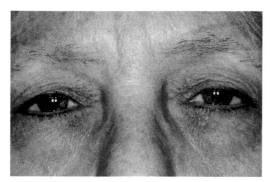

Fig. 5. It is important to diagnose any underlying ptosis during the preoperative evaluation, as in this patient who presents with evidence of bilateral upper eyelid ptosis and dermatochalasis.

Box 3
Preoperative identification of high-risk patients
1. Dry eye syndrome/Sjögren syndrome
2. Thyroid disease
3. Lower lid laxity
4. Negative vector
5. Scleral show
6. Previous facial trauma
7. Previous facial surgery
8. Psychological issues
9. Unrealistic expectations

with raising the lower lid, there is evidence of lower lid retraction (**Fig. 10**). The development of lower lid retraction from postsurgical manipulation is characterized by inflammation, scarring, shortening, and cicatricial tethering of the middle and posterior lamella. Examination in this region should also include any evidence of lower lid hollowing, which can be managed with the use of dermal soft tissue augmentation; hyaluronic acid is the preferred dermal filler in this region. Many of the issues described earlier can be diagnosed and addressed before or during lower eyelid blepharoplasty.

DRY EYE SYNDROME/OCULAR IRRITATION

Patients present with ocular irritation from multiple causes, including dry eye syndrome, lower eyelid malposition, lid retraction, lagophthalmos, blepharitis, and alterations in the tear film and/or blink reflex. Dry eye syndrome affects up to 17% of women and up to 12% of men in the general population, and so it is imperative to diagnose and treat this condition before surgery, because the incidence of dry eye syndrome following blepharoplasty is between 8% and 21%.[11–14]

Ocular surface lubrication can be influenced by quantitative deficiencies such as decreased tear production, qualitative problems in the mucous and lipid layers of the tear film from blepharitis/meibomitis, and also from tear distribution problems secondary to a poor blink mechanism, or from a combination of all of these factors. Dry eye symptoms include discomfort, dryness, burning, stinging, foreign-body sensation, gritty feeling, blurry vision, photophobia, itching, and redness. Risk factors for dry eyes include underlying systemic disease, menopause, previous lid surgery, and history of laser-assisted in situ keratomileusis (LASIK).[15] Preoperatively, patients should be assessed for possible dry eye syndrome with a Schirmer test. The Schirmer strip is inserted in the lower eyelid at the lateral limbus after a topical anesthetic drop has been inserted into the eye (**Fig. 11**). After 5 minutes, the Schirmer strip is removed and a measurement is recorded; normal measurements are between 10 and 15 mm of wetting. If the measurement is significantly

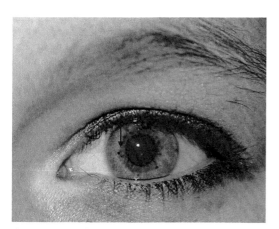

Fig. 6. Patient showing a normal MRD1.

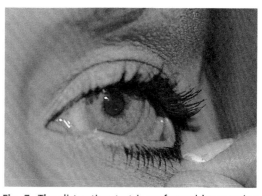

Fig. 7. The distraction test is performed by grasping the eyelid and pulling anteriorly; if the distracted distance is greater than 6 to 8 mm, then lower lid laxity is evident.

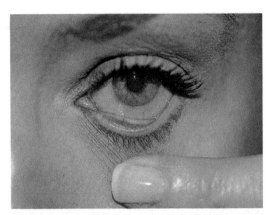

Fig. 8. The snap back test, which is used to assess the function of the orbicularis oculi muscle and the amount of lower eyelid tone, is accomplished by displacing the lower eyelid toward the orbital rim and releasing the lid. Slow return of the lower eyelid reveals decreased lid tone.

less than 10 mm, then the patient has evidence of hyposecretion of tears with dry eye syndrome. Although the results of Schirmer testing may be inconsistent, the test is beneficial for documenting evidence of severe dry eyes. With cosmetic blepharoplasty, patients with dry eye syndrome may experience worsening of their condition, and in severe cases it may even be a contraindication to surgery.

Saadat and Drenser[16] discussed that by preserving the orbicularis muscle and its innervation, blepharoplasty could be safely performed in patients with dry eyes. The dynamics of eyelid closure, including tear pumping and tear distribution, are not affected with preservation of the orbicularis muscle and its innervation. Fagien[17] noted not only the importance of the preservation of the orbicularis muscle from a functional standpoint but also for improved cosmetic results by retaining a youthful fullness to the upper eyelid region. Cosmetic surgeons must be aware of the

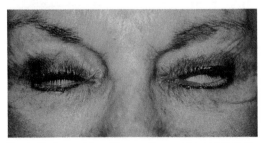

Fig. 9. Patient with evidence of severe lagophthalmos secondary to severe upper and lower eyelid retraction following overaggressive upper and lower lid blepharoplasty.

long-term implications of lid surgery from an aesthetic and functional standpoint to assure correct lid position and closure for adequate corneal protection and ocular lubrication.

Normal tearing is divided into 3 components:

1. Production and release of tears from the lacrimal gland and accessory glands
2. Blinking and distribution of tears
3. Tear pumping into the lacrimal drainage system.

As discussed earlier, the action of the orbicularis muscle is responsible for the second 2 components.[16] With preservation of the orbicularis muscle and its innervations in transconjunctival lower lid blepharoplasty, there is a decreased incidence of complications of retraction, scleral show, and lacrimal pump problems compared with the external skin-muscle flap technique. Hester and colleagues[10] recommended eliminating trauma to the orbital septum lower lid during blepharoplasty by avoiding the plane between the orbicularis muscle. When performing transconjunctival lower lid blepharoplasty, either a pinch technique or laser resurfacing can be used to address lower lid rhytids.

ORBITAL HEMORRHAGE

The most feared complication of periocular surgery is loss of vision or even blindness secondary to orbital hemorrhage. The risk of orbital hemorrhage is 1 in 2000 and the risk of orbital hemorrhage with visual loss is 1 in 10,000.[18] During the preoperative evaluation, patients' risk factors should be identified to decrease the risk of this devastating outcome. Included among risk factors for orbital hemorrhage are antiplatelet or anticoagulant medications (including homeopathic or herbal medications), history of hypertension, and history of abnormal bruising or bleeding or underlying disease that may contribute to bleeding.[18,19] It is important to obtain a complete history of the patient's medications, including vitamins and herbs, which affect coagulation. Preoperatively, patients should be instructed to discontinue Coumadin, aspirin, nonsteroidal antiinflammatory drugs (NSAIDs), vitamin E, omega-3 fatty acids, garlic, and other supplements or herbs with blood-thinning effects. The patient should also be provided with a list of medications that affect coagulation; the author's surgical counselor periodically updates this list (Fig. 12). Many surgeons also recommend having patients take *Arnica montana*, vitamin K, and bromelain in an attempt to limit postoperative edema and ecchymoses.

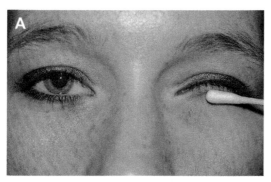

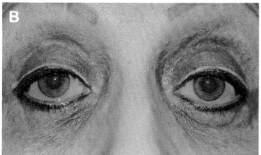

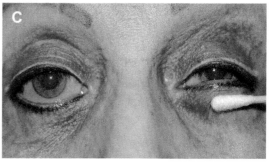

Fig. 10. Defined as inferior malposition of the lower eyelid margin without eyelid eversion, lower eyelid retraction is assessed by placing upward traction on the lower eyelid. (*A*) In normal conditions, the lower lid can be displaced to the midpupil or above. (*B*). Patient with postoperative lower eyelid retraction with evidence of scleral show, lateral canthal dystopia, and periorbital hollowing. (*C*) The same patient as in (*B*) has evidence of lid retraction, therefore the vertical displacement of the lid with manual raising is restricted.

Haas and colleagues[18] found comorbidities of orbital hemorrhage included past history of hypertension, preoperative aspirin intake, postoperative vomiting, and postoperative physical activity. These investigators also noted an increased risk

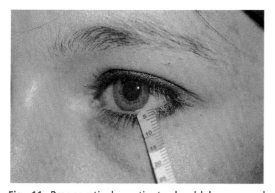

Fig. 11. Preoperatively, patients should be assessed for possible dry eye syndrome with a Schirmer test, with the strip inserted at the lateral limbus after the use of a topical anesthetic. After 5 minutes, the Schirmer strip is removed; normal range is between 10 and 15 mm. If the measurement is significantly less than 10 mm, then the patient has evidence of hyposecretion of tears with possible dry eye syndrome.

of orbital hemorrhage during the first 3 hours following surgery, with the risk decreasing 24 hours after surgery, although Teng and colleagues[20] reported a patient who presented with an orbital hemorrhage 9 days following a cosmetic blepharoplasty that resulted in permanent visual loss.[18]

Intraoperatively, emphasis should be directed to controlling the blood pressure to decrease the risks of bleeding. Secondary to the vasodilation effects from general anesthesia, local anesthesia is preferred. To achieve the maximum vasoconstrictive effects of epinephrine after the administration of local anesthesia, it is important to wait at least 15 minutes before starting surgery. Meticulous dissection of the orbital fat pads is important to avoid traction and decrease the risk of posterior orbital bleeding, with particular attention to cauterization of any pinpoint areas of bleeding from the orbicularis muscle before skin closure.

Orbital hemorrhage in the postoperative period is the leading cause of visual loss from cosmetic eyelid surgery, therefore early detection and treatment are critical.[21–27] Postoperative checking of vision is recommended and patients should be encouraged to call their physician immediately with any signs of decreased vision, pain, or rapidly

PLEASE AVOID THESE MEDICATIONS FOR AT LEAST 10 DAYS BEFORE SURGERY
Orally Administered medications That Increase Bleeding Time
Preparations that contain nonsteroidal anti-inflammatory agents

Aches-N-Pain (ibuprofen)
Actiprofen (ibuprofen)
Actron (ketoprofen)
Addaprin (ibuprofen)
Advil (ibuprofen)
Advil Cold & Sinus
(ibuprofen)
Aleve (naproxen sodium)
Anaprox (naproxen sodium)
Anaprox DS (naproxen
sodium)
Ansaid (flurbiprofen)
APO-Diclo (diclofenac)
APO-Diflunisal (diflunisal)
APO-Flurbiprofen (flurbiprofen)
APO-Ibuprofen (ibuprofen)
APO-Indomethacin
(indomethacin)
APO-Keto (ketoprofen)
APO-Napro (naproxen)
APO-Napro-Na (naproxen
sodium)
APO-Naproxen (naproxen)
APO-Piroxicam (piroxicam)
APO-Sulin (sulindac)
Bayer Select (ibuprofen)
Butazolidin (phenylbutazone)
Cataflam (diclofenac)
Clinoril (sulindac)
CoAdvil (ibuprofen)
Cotylbutazone (phenylbuazone)
Cramp End (ibuprofen)
Daypro (oxaprozin)
Diclofenac
Diflunisal
Dimetapp Sinus (ibuprofen)
Dolgesic (ibuprofen)
Dolobid (diflunisal)
Dristan Sinus (ibuprofen)
EC-Naprosyn (naproxen)
Etodolac
Excedrin IB (ibuprofen)
Feldene (piroxicam)
Fenoprofen
Flurbiprofen
Froben (flurbiprofen)
Genpril (ibuprofen)
Haltran (ibuprofen)

Ibifon 600 (ibuprofen)
Ibren (ibuprofen
IBU (ibuprofen)
Ibu 200 (ibuprofen)
Ibu 400 (ibuprofen)
Ibu 600 (ibuprofen)
Ibu 800 (ibuprofen)
Ibuprin (ibuprofen)
Ibuprofen
Ibuprohm (ibuprofen)
IBU-TAB (ibuprofen)
Indochron ER
(indomethacin)
Indocid (indomethacin)
Indocin (indomethacin)
Indomethacin
ketoprofen
Lodine (etodolac)
meclofenamate
Meclomen (meclofenamate)
Medipren (ibuprofen)
Menadol (ibuprofen)
Midol 200 (ibuprofen)
Midol IB (ibuprofen)
Mobic
Motrin (ibuprofen)
Motrin IB (ibuprofen)
Motrin IB Sinus (ibuprofen)
Nalfon (fenoprofen calcium)
Naprelan (naproxen)
Napron X (naproxen)
Naprosyn (naproxen)
Naprosyn E (naproxen)
Naprosyn SR (naproxen)
naproxen
naproxen sodium
Naxen (Naproxen)
Novo-Difenac (diclofenac)
Novo-Diflunisl (diflunisal)
Novo-Flurprofen
(flurbiprofen)
Novo-Keto-EC (ketoprofen)
Novo-Methacin
(indomethacin)
Novo-Naprox (naproxen)
Novo-Naprox Sodium
(naprosen sodium)
Novo-Pirocam (piroxicam)

Novo-Profen (ibuprofen)
Novo-Sundac (sulindac)
Novo-Tolmetin (tolmetin)
Nu-Diclo (diclofenac)
Nu-Flubiprofen
(flurbiprofen)
Nu-Ibuprofen (ibuprofen)
Nu-Indo (indomethacin)
Nu-Naprox (naproxen)
Nu-Pirox (piroxicam)
Nuprin (ibuprofen)
Nu-Sulindac (sulindac)
Orudis (ketoprofen)
Orudis E (ketoprofen)
Orudis KT(ketoprofen)
Orudis SR (ketoprofen)
Oruvail (ketoprofen)
Pamprin-IB (ibuprofen)
PediaProfen(ibuprofen)
Piroxicam
Ponstan (mefenamic acid)
Ponstel (mefenamic acid)
Q-Profen (ibuprofen)
Relafen (nabumetone)
Rhodis (ketoprofen)
Rufen (ibuprofen)
Saleto-200 (ibuprofen)
Saleto-400 (ibuprofen)
Saleto-600 (ibuprofen)
Saleto-800 (ibuprofen)
Sine-Aid IB (ibuprofen)
sulindac
Synflex (naproxen)
Synflex SR (naproxen)
Tolectin (tolemetin
sodium)
tolmentin
Toradol (ketorolac)
Trendar (ibuprofen)
Ulraprin (ibuprofen)
Unipro (ibuprofen)
Valprin (ibuprofen)
Voltaren (diclofenac)
Voltaren Rapide
(diclofenac)
Voltaren SR (diclofenac)

• Tylenol (Acetaminophen), Celebrex (celecoxib), and Vioxx (rofecoxib) are permissible because they do not interfere with clotting.
Please avoid Vitamin E, garlic, ginger, ginkgo, and ginseng for at least 10 days before surgery as well.

Fig. 12. List of medications that can result in blood thinning, including over-the-counter medications, that patients are encouraged to discontinue preoperatively before their periocular cosmetic surgery.

PLEASE AVOID THESE MEDICATIONS FOR AT LEAST 10 DAYS BEFORE SURGERY
Orally Administered medications That Increase Bleeding Time
Preparations that contain nonsteroidal anti-inflammatory agents

217	Damason-P	Neogesic
217 Strong	Darvon compound	Nervine
4-Way Cold tablets	Darvon compound-65	Night-time Effervescent cold tablets
Acuprin 81 (aspirin)	Darvon with ASA	Norgesic
Adult Analgestic pain reliever	Darvon-N with ASA	Norgesic Forte
Aggrenox	Dasin	Norwich extra-strength aspirin
Alka-Seltzer	Dolcin	Novasen)
Anacin	Dolomine	Orphenagesic
Analval	Dolprn #3 tablets	Orphenagesic Forte
Anodynos	Drinophen	Oxycodone and aspirin
Antidol	Duradyne	P-A-C
APAC Improved	Easprin	Pain Aid
APO-ASA	Ecotrin	Pain reliever tablets
APO-ASEN	Emagrin	Panodynes
Arco Pain	Empirin	Pepto-Bismol
Arthrisin	Empirin with codeine	Percodan
Arthritis Pain Formula	Entrophen	Percodan-Demi
Artria SR	Equagesic	Persistin
ASA	Equazine-M	Phenetron compound
Ascriptin	Excedrin	PMS with ASA
Aspercin	Fiogesic tablets	Presalin
Aspergum	Fiorgen PF	Propoxyphen compound
Aspermin	Fiorinal	Propoxyphen napsylate with ASA
Asprin	Fiorinal with codeine	Quiet World tablets
Aspirin with codeine	Gelpirin tablets	Rhinoceps
Aspir-Low	Gemnisyn	Robaxisal tablets
Aspir-Tab	Genaced	Roxiprin
Aspirtab Max	Genacote	Roxiprin tablets
Astone	Genprin	Salabuff
Astrin	Gensan	Salatin
Axotal	Goody's extra strength	Saleto
Azdone tablets	Goody's Headache powder	Salocol
B-A-C tablets	Halfprin	Sine-Off sinus medicine tablets
Bayer Aspirin	Headache tablet	Sloprin
Bayer children's cold tablets	Heathprin	Soma compound tablets
BC powder	Herbopyrine	Soma compound with codeine
BC Tablets	Instantine	St. Joseph
Buffaprin	Isollyl Improved	Stanback powder
Buffasal	Kalmex	Supac
Bufferin	Lanorinal	Synalgos-DC capsules
Buffets II	Lortab with ASA	Talwin compound
Buffex	Magnaprin	Tenol-Plus
Buffinol	Marnal	Trigesic
C2	Measurin	Tri-Pain
Calamine	Micrainin	Ursinus Inlay-Tabs
Cama arthritis pain reliever	Meprobamate and aspirin	Valesin
Carisoprodol compound tablets	Meprogesic Q	Vanquish
Children's aspirin	Midol for cramps,maximum strength	Verin
Cope	Midol Original	Wesprin Buffered
Coryphen	Momentum muscular backache formula	Zorprin

• Tylenol (Acetaminophen), Celebrex (celecoxib), and Vioxx (rofecoxib) are permissible because they do not interfere with clotting.
Please avoid Vitamin E, garlic, ginger, ginkgo, and ginseng for at least 10 days before surgery as well.

Fig. 12. (*continued*)

increasing edema. Physicians should be available to see patients in a timely fashion if patients experience any of the signs or symptoms described earlier. Patients are encouraged to avoid bending, lifting, and straining; they should rest with their head elevated and ice packs should be applied for 30 minutes every hour while the patient is awake for the initial 2 to 3 days following surgery.

INFECTION

The risk of postoperative infection following periocular surgery is low secondary to the rich vascular supply of the eyelids. Carter and colleagues[28] reported the infection rate at 0.2% in patients who had undergone upper or lower blepharoplasty without laser resurfacing and slightly higher at 0.4% in patients who had adjunctive laser resurfacing in addition to blepharoplasty. Postoperative infections typically present between 4 and 7 days after surgery.[28] Carter and colleagues[28] recommend the routine use of topical antibiotic ointment as a sufficient postoperative treatment regimen for patients undergoing blepharoplasty without the need for prophylactic systemic antibiotics.

PERIOCULAR LASER RESURFACING

Complications related to periocular laser resurfacing include scarring, hyperpigmentation, hypopigmentation, long-lasting erythema, and infection. A prophylactic antibacterial and antiviral systemic regimen is typically initiated a few days before the procedure and continued for 1 week postoperatively. Intraoperatively, feathering of the laser passes is recommended between treated and untreated areas to limit possible demarcation lines. Conservative treatment with laser resurfacing is also recommended along the angle of the mandible because this area can scar easily.

Postoperative wound care is focused on resolution of erythema, avoiding infections, and limiting postinflammatory hyperpigmentation. Topical applications of Aquaphor or Vaseline combined with hydrocortisone 1% cream and dilute cool solutions vinegar soaks are used during the postoperative period. Sun protection is recommended with sunscreen with a sun protection factor of 30 or greater following the laser treatment, and postoperative hyperpigmentation can be treated with Hydroquinone 4% cream as necessary.

LASIK

Patients seeking cosmetic eyelid surgery are in the same age demographic as patients who are interested in undergoing LASIK surgery. For patients who have undergone previous LASIK surgery, it is important to emphasize the increased risk of postoperative dry eye syndrome following cosmetic periocular surgery. According to the American Society of Cataract and Refractive Surgery, patients who undergo LASIK surgery have a 15% to 25% chance of developing dry eyes during the postoperative period from a transient neurotrophic keratopathy secondary to severing of corneal nerves during LASIK surgery.[29] With LASIK the corneal nerves, which enter the midstroma and run centrally, are severed and must regenerate. The deeper the ablation with the LASIK surgery, the greater the distance the surgically amputated nerve trunks need to regenerate to reinervate the cornea.

The normal corneal reflex arc is triggered by ocular irritation or foreign-body sensation, which causes ocular surface desiccation, leading to the blink reflex, which sweeps the cornea with tears. After blepharoplasty, patients have a transient lagophthalmos, but the corneal reflex arc blinking pattern is increased to prevent dry eye symptoms. The challenge with LASIK surgery is that the corneal sensory nerves are transected and the normal blink reflex is blunted, which results in decreased corneal sensitivity and a decreased blink rate, thus resulting in decreased tear production.[29] The combination of LASIK and blepharoplasty can further increase the risk of severe dry eye condition.

According to Shoja and Besharati,[30] the risk of dry eye syndrome after LASIK surgery is increased in patients with higher degrees of myopia preoperatively, in patients treated to a greater ablation depth, and also in female patients. De Paiva and colleagues[31] also noted a correlation between the risk of dry eye syndrome and the degree of myopia preoperatively, whereas Albietz and colleagues[32] found an increased risk of dry eye syndrome in the Asian population. Michaeli and colleagues[33] found evidence of decreased corneal sensitivity and decreased Schirmer testing following LASIK, with return to normal levels after 3 months. Korn and colleagues[34] developed an algorithm for the workup and possible treatment of patients with a history of previous LASIK who are planning to undergo blepharoplasty. It may be prudent to perform the blepharoplasty before LASIK surgery, because there may be an astigmatic change in the refraction by relieving the weight of the upper lid on the cornea.

BOTOX COSMETIC

Cosmetic surgeons must be aware that the widespread use of Botox Cosmetic in our patient demographic can affect surgical planning. Patients should be questioned regarding previous use of Botox Cosmetic, particularly the specific treated area and whether the patient will continue the use of Botox Cosmetic following the planned surgery. Botox Cosmetic can also be used preoperatively to augment surgical results, such as in treating the brow depressors (corrugators, procerus, and lateral orbicularis oculi) 1 to 2 weeks before a patient undergoes endoscopic brow lift surgery to decrease the action of the brow depressors during the postoperative period. Brow asymmetry can also be improved by the selective administration of Botox Cosmetic into the brow elevators (frontalis muscle) to lower brow position and in the lateral brow depressors (orbicularis oculi) to raise brow position as needed **(Fig. 13)**.[35,36] Selective use of Botox Cosmetic can also treat minimal to moderate ptosis by performing subdermal injections in the pretarsal orbicularis oculi at the extreme medial and lateral areas of the upper eyelid.[37]

Migration of Botox Cosmetic injections into facial regions in close proximity to intended injection sites can result in unwanted side effects, such as ptosis, which occurs from migration of the botulinum A exotoxin from periocular sites through the orbital septum to the levator muscle of the upper eyelid. The cosmetic surgeon can treat this complication of secondary ptosis with the administration of Apraclonidine 0.5%, a selective α-2-adrenergic agonist, Alphagan or Naphcon. The resultant contraction of the Müller muscle results in an elevation of 1 to 2 mm in the lid height.[38,39] In addition to lid ptosis, other possible complications of Botox Cosmetic treatments include diplopia, lower lid ectropion, eyebrow ptosis, and asymmetrical results. It is recommended to avoid Botox Cosmetic injections during facial surgical procedures secondary to the possible risk of diffusion. Injections in the crow's feet region should be subcutaneous to avoid the risk of bruising from the orbicularis oculi muscle. Any bruising noted during the administration of Botox Cosmetic should be treated with direct immediate pressure to the site.

CHEMOSIS

Defined as transudative edema of the bulbar and/or palpebral conjunctiva, chemosis is evident as visible yellowish or pink swelling of the conjunctiva.[40] Postoperative chemosis presents with foreign-body sensation, epiphora, irritation, pain, redness, and blurred vision. Causes of postoperative chemosis are multifactorial and include exposure, prolonged postoperative inflammation, periorbital and facial edema, extensive conjunctival manipulation, and postoperative disruption/dysfunction of the lymphatic system.[40–43] The lateral half of the eyelid lymphatic system drains to the preauricular node and the medial half drains to the submandibular node, thus periorbital and facial edema cause secondary regional lymphatic stasis that can trigger and cause worsening of chemosis.[40] Lymphatic dysfunction occurs secondarily to structural damage that occurs during surgery to the lymphatic channels that drain the conjunctiva.[40,44]

Weinfeld and colleagues[40] divided the presentation of chemosis into 4 categories, with the treatment protocol dictated by the category, and also noted predisposing factors for the development of chemosis to include increased surgical time, resulting in increased periorbital swelling and exposure of the conjunctiva and lagophthalmos from upper eyelid blepharoplasty and/or brow lift. For most patients, the presence of chemosis resolves spontaneously during the early postoperative period, but in some instances, a combination of pharmacologic, mechanical, and/or surgical therapies may be necessary. The cosmetic surgeon should focus on the importance of prevention of chemosis by minimizing intraoperative risk factors with appropriate timely therapeutic intervention for persistent chemosis noted during the postoperative period.[40]

STRABISMUS/DIPLOPIA

Transient diplopia, which may occur postoperatively secondary to the effects of local anesthesia or orbital edema, is self-limited. Permanent diplopia is usually secondary to damage to either the inferior or superior oblique muscles or inferior rectus muscle during fat excision.[7,45] Putterman[46]

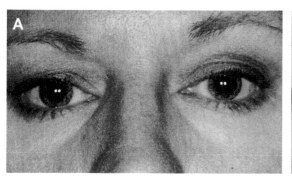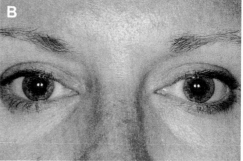

Fig. 13. Botox Cosmetic to address brow asymmetry (*A*) Patient with evidence of brow asymmetry; left higher than right. (*B*) Same patient following the use of Botox Cosmetic to selectively lower the left brow and raise the raise brow combined with upper eyelid blepharoplasty.

described strabismus after cosmetic blepharoplasty secondary to restrictive changes from scar formation, particularly from excision of the temporal lower eyelid fat pad. The risk of diplopia can be decreased during lower lid blepharoplasty by identifying and avoiding the inferior oblique muscle as it courses between the medial and central lower eyelid fat compartments.[47] Nonresolving diplopia following blepharoplasty may require strabismus surgery if the patient remains symptomatic.

TREATMENT OF COMPLICATIONS

What is the typical presentation of the unhappy patient after blepharoplasty? There are 3 major areas of concern for a patient who has problems following a cosmetic blepharoplasty:

1. Uncomfortable/symptomatic issues
2. Cosmetic issues and functional issues
3. Combination of (1) and (2).

Cosmetic issues include asymmetry, periorbital hollowing, deep superior sulcus, alteration of the lid crease/fold, lateral canthal dystopia, eyelid malposition, ptosis, and unnatural appearance. Patients may have functional problems including scleral show with corneal exposure lid laxity, chemosis, lagophthalmos, and retraction. In addition to cosmetic and functional concerns, patients may also experience symptoms such as discomfort, burning, stinging, dry eye/foreign-body sensation, blurry vision, photophobia, itching, and redness.

ORBITAL HEMORRHAGE MANAGEMENT

Because orbital hemorrhage is the leading cause of visual loss from cosmetic eyelid surgery, patients should be instructed to contact their surgeon immediately with any evidence of visual loss, pain, diplopia, or rapidly increasing edema, because early detection and treatment are critical (**Box 4**).[21–27] Physicians should be available to see patients in a timely fashion if patients experience any of these signs or symptoms, and patients should be examined for evidence of visual loss, proptosis, relative afferent pupillary defect, and/ or limited extraocular motility (**Fig. 14**). The goal of the treatment of orbital hemorrhage is to decrease the orbital pressure and restore blood flow to the eye. The wound should be opened to identify any active bleeding sites followed by lateral canthotomy and cantholysis to completely free the lower eyelid, with careful attention to lyse any eyelid adhesions to the orbital rim. Once it is determined that the lower lid is freely mobile, any active bleeding sites should be cauterized, and any hematomas should be drained. Rarely, orbital decompression may be necessary. A tapering dose of systemic steroids can be initiated and an ocular examination, including measurement of the intraocular pressure and assessment of retinal perfusion, should be performed by an ophthalmologist. If increased intraocular pressure is noted, the ophthalmologist may initiate a treatment regimen of topical or oral glaucoma agents. Following drainage of an orbital hemorrhage, the patient should elevate the head of the bed when sleeping and should be carefully monitored for visual acuity, pupil examination, intraocular pressure, and examination of the fundus.[48]

UPPER EYELID BLEPHAROPLASTY/BROW SURGERY

With upper eyelid blepharoplasty, surgeons should focus on conservative upper eyelid skin removal, with careful attention to reestablishing the upper eyelid crease, with an aesthetically pleasing result. Regarding the amount of skin excision in upper eyelid blepharoplasty, one should keep in mind the Flower rule of preserving at least 20 mm of upper eyelid skin for normal lid function.[49] Included in the evaluation is the assessment

---

Box 4
Orbital hemorrhage warning signs/symptoms

1. Orbital pain
2. Loss of vision
3. Proptosis
4. Relative afferent pupillary defect
5. Limited extraocular motility
6. Increased orbital pressure/tense orbit

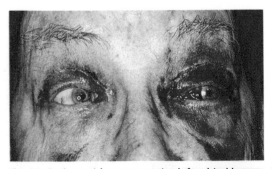

Fig. 14. Patient with postoperative left orbital hemorrhage with evidence of proptosis, relative afferent pupillary defect, and limited extraocular motility (see **Fig. 11**).

for underlying brow ptosis and/or lid ptosis, which can be surgically repaired at the same time as the planned blepharoplasty (**Figs. 15** and **16**). Possible complications of endoscopic brow surgery include alopecia, numbness, facial nerve injury, and asymmetry. Meticulous attention to operating in the correct tissue plane during surgery, with limited electrocautery of the wound during closure, is paramount to achieving superior aesthetic results in endoscopic brow lift surgery.

Careful attention to the upper eyelid crease in blepharoplasty is necessary to achieve a natural contour, therefore upper eyelids should be assessed for asymmetry of the lid crease/fold. The treatment of asymmetrical lid crease may prove to be a challenge for the surgeon, particularly if the crease is too high. It is more difficult to lower a high crease, which may be secondary to excessive fat removal, which leads to extra skin that fills in the iatrogenic concavity. A low crease can be easier to raise with the use of supratarsal fixation. A soft upper eyelid crease can be formed with a 3-point suture by taking a bite through the lower portion of the skin/orbicularis muscle incision, then a bite through levator aponeurosis, and then exiting through the upper portion of the skin/orbicularis muscle incision.

The presence of lacrimal gland prolapse can often be noted more easily during the surgery as the lacrimal gland is a firm, fibrous gray structure compared with the soft, yellowish orbital fat. If lacrimal gland prolapse is diagnosed, then resuspension to the periosteum of the superior orbital rim is recommended to alleviate this problem.[50,51] Medial canthal webbing results from either an improperly placed incision or excessive skin removal. This complication can be avoided by angling the incision slightly superior at the medial extent of the upper lid blepharoplasty incision and not extending the incision past the level of the superior punctum. Treatment includes massage initially, and if complete resolution is not observed, then a Z-plasty may be considered.

PTOSIS SURGERY

Intraoperatively, eyelids should also be evaluated for any evidence of ptosis with underlying levator dehiscence; correction should be performed at that time. It is imperative for the surgeon who performs cosmetic eyelid surgery to be aware of the close proximity of the levator aponeurosis to the inferior blepharoplasty incision to avoid damage, because the levator aponeurosis attaches to the orbicularis muscle/skin at this point. If the inferior upper lid blepharoplasty incision is too deep, then dehiscence of the levator aponeurosis can result.[52] In addition, orbital septal incisions to gain access to the preaponeurotic fat pads should be made near the superior lip of the wound while tenting the orbital septum 90° from the levator aponeurosis to further decrease the risk of iatrogenic damage to the levator aponeurosis.

Patients who present with ptosis after blepharoplasty may have multiple causes, including unrecognized preoperative ptosis, direct levator damage, stretching of the levator, and tethering secondary to the orbital septum being inadvertently incorporated into the closure of the lid. Surgical intervention in the postoperative period includes standard ptosis surgery such as levator advancement or the Müller muscle-conjunctival resection procedure.[53,54] In levator advancement repair, the central anterior tarsus should be exposed, with placement of the suture in the central 5 mm of the tarsus. The suture should be placed in the upper third of the tarsus because lower placement may result in ectropion of the upper lid (**Fig. 17**). It is also

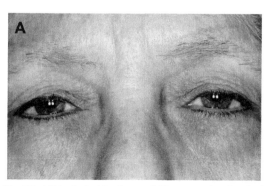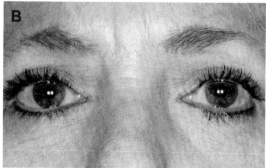

Fig. 15. (*A*) Included in the eyelid/brow evaluation is the assessment for underlying lid ptosis, which is evident in addition to dermatochalasis in this female patient. (*B*) Same patient following combined bilateral upper eyelid blepharoplasty and upper eyelid levator advancement.

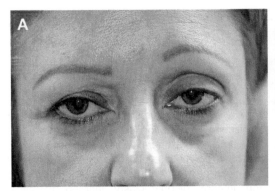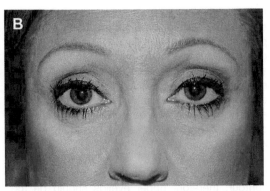

Fig. 16. (*A*) Included in the eyelid/brow evaluation is the assessment for underlying brow ptosis and lid ptosis, which is evident in addition to dermatochalasis in this female patient. (*B*) Same patient following combined brow and eyelid surgery.

recommended that the position of the upper eyelid be verified in the sitting position during surgery before permanently tying the sutures. The use of nonreactive permanent sutures for eyelid closure may result in decreased rates of scarring, epithelial suture cysts, and milia.

MANAGEMENT OF UPPER EYELID RETRACTION/LAGOPHTHALMOS

Upper eyelid retraction can occur from anterior lamellar deficiency, tethering of the orbital septum, or secondary to a combination of the two. Anterior lamellar deficiency, diagnosed when the lagophthalmos resolves when the brows are manually placed inferiorly, may require a full-thickness skin graft for surgical correction if the patient does

not improve with massage. Upper eyelid tethering, which is an outcome from incorporation of the orbital septum into the eyelid closure, results in normal eyelid position in primary gaze, but with evidence of lid lag in down gaze and lagophthalmos that does not improve when the brows are manually placed inferiorly. Correction of upper eyelid tethering requires opening the wound to isolate and release the incorporated orbital septum, which is more easily accomplished during the early postoperative period to decrease the risk of anterior lamellar contraction.

MANAGEMENT OF DEEP SUPERIOR SULCUS

The degree of deepness of the superior sulcus is determined by the interplay between the brow

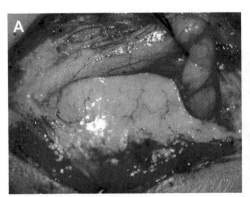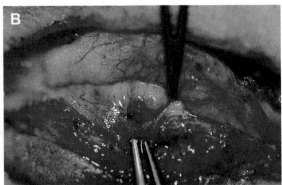

Fig. 17. (*A*) During levator advancement, it is important to dissect and enter the orbital septum superiorly to avoid the close attachment of the levator lower incision. (*B*) In levator advancement repair, the central anterior tarsus should be exposed, with placement of the suture in the central 5 mm of the tarsus and in the upper one-third of the tarsus, because lower placement may result in ectropion. The author also recommends that the position of the upper eyelid be verified in the sitting position during surgery before permanently tying the sutures.

fat, preaponeurotic fat pads, orbital septum, and the levator aponeurosis. Cosmetic surgeons should strive for a natural brow contour and full upper eyelid sulcus, with an emphasis on avoiding the creation of a lid crease that is too high, to avoid a deep superior sulcus. Treatment options to correct the deep superior sulcus include ptosis repair, reposition of fat, altering brow position with Botox Cosmetic, fat grafts, and placement of filler material or dermis fat graft to add volume.

MANAGEMENT OF LOWER LID HOLLOWING

Postoperative lower eyelid periorbital hollowing is another common complication that can occur following aggressive lower lid blepharoplasty or can be secondary to aging changes related to soft-tissue atrophy, thinning of the skin, soft-tissue descent, and/or orbital fat herniation cephalad to this area.[55,56] Autologous fat can be injected or orbital fat can be transposed to add volume and correct the tear trough deformity.[55,56] Dermal facial fillers such as hyaluronic acid can be injected into this region for volume replacement to mask underlying hollowing.[57–60] Treatment is recommended in a deeper, supraperiosteal plane to reduce visibility of the product in this area of thin tissue.[57]

Patients may benefit from discontinuing all blood-thinning agents before undergoing facial dermal filler procedures. If hyaluronic acid fillers are injected too superficially, a bluish color may occur secondary to the Tyndall effect. This complication can be treated by nicking the papule with a number 11 blade or with the administration of hyaluronidase.[55] The latter treatment can also be used to treat areas of irregularity or asymmetry. It is recommended to have nitropaste available for the treatment of any vascular compromise noted during treatments. Following facial filler applications, it is recommended that patients limit massaging in the treated areas and apply ice packs to limit edema and ecchymoses. The combined use of Botox Cosmetic and dermal fillers may lead to improved aesthetic results.

MANAGEMENT OF CHEMOSIS

Causes of postoperative chemosis are multifactorial and include exposure, prolonged postoperative inflammation, periorbital edema, extensive conjunctival manipulation, and postoperative disruption of the lymphatic system.[40–43] Intraoperative recommendations to decrease the risk of chemosis include limited dissection, frequent ocular lubrication during the surgery, intermittent forced eyelid closure, and the use of a temporary tarsorrhaphy suture.[40] Treatment of postoperative chemosis consists of medical therapies, with possible mechanical and surgical modalities if necessary. Initial treatment should consist of lubrication, topical steroids, head elevation, and eye patching.[40] If resolution of the chemosis is not complete, then drainage conjunctivotomy and temporary tarsorrhaphy may be used.[40,41] Putterman[61] advocates the use of patient finger compression of the eyelid over the area of chemosis. The compression is accomplished 4 to 10 times per day as necessary at the patient elevates the lower eyelid over the chemotic area and applies pressure for approximately 10 seconds (see **Fig. 15**).[61]

MANAGEMENT OF DRY EYE SYNDROME/ OCULAR IRRITATION

Dry eye symptoms include discomfort, dryness, burning, stinging, foreign-body sensation, gritty feeling, blurry vision, photophobia, itching, and redness. Surgeons who perform blepharoplasty should strive to diagnose dry eyes preoperatively and maximize comfort through various treatment options.[12] Ocular surface lubrication can be influenced by quantitative deficiencies such as decreased tear production, qualitative problems in the mucous and lipid layers of the tear film from blepharitis/meibomitis, which lead to evaporation of the tear film, and also from tear distribution problems secondary to a poor blink mechanism, or from a combination of all of these factors.

The treatment of preexisting ocular surface problems includes medical and surgical options. The following medical options can be used to treat dry eye syndrome and reduce ocular irritation: lubrication (artificial tears/ointment), topical steroids, NSAIDs, topical cyclosporine (Restasis), and collage/silicone punctual plugs. The treatment of blepharitis/meibomitis includes the use of doxycycline, flax seed oil, omega-3 fatty acids, and warm compresses/scrubs. These options can also be initiated in the preoperative period for patients who have planned revision surgery. Other preexisting conditions mentioned earlier can be corrected during the surgical procedure, including lid malposition, lid laxity, and lid retraction.

MANAGEMENT OF LOWER EYELID RETRACTION/ECTROPION/LAGOPHTHALMOS

The most common complications of cosmetic lower eyelid blepharoplasty are retraction, dry eyes, scleral show, lagophthalmos, lateral canthal dystopia, periorbital hollowing, and ectropion.

Defined as inferior malposition of the lower eyelid margin without eyelid eversion, lower eyelid retraction is assessed by placing upward traction on the lower eyelid. Signs of lid retraction include scleral show, round sad eyes, lateral canthal rounding, corneal exposure, loss of the almond-shaped eye, and lagophthalmos. Lid retraction, which develops from postsurgical manipulation, is characterized by inflammation, scarring, short-ening, and cicatricial tethering of the middle and posterior lamella (**Fig. 18**). Dense scarring occurs between the orbital septum and orbital fat, with secondary adhesions to the orbicularis muscle, which results in tethering of the eyelid as the orbital septum is attached to the orbital rim. The vertical contraction of the eyelid results in hollowing as the lower lid fat is pushed posteriorly into the orbit. With lower lid retraction the skin moves easily, but the tarsus is tethered in place. In a normal eyelid, the lateral canthal complex moves medially with eyelid closure, but with evidence of lower lid retraction, this movement may be decreased or even completely absent.

Excessive skin excision during a transcuta-neous blepharoplasty can result in anterior lamellar deficiency and ectropion, which is defined as an eyelid malposition in which the lid margin is everted from the normal apposition to the globe. A transcutaneous incisional approach results in skin contraction of 2 to 3 mm, even without the removal of any skin, secondary to scarring and tightening along the dissection plane between the orbicularis muscle and the orbital septum.[62] The development of

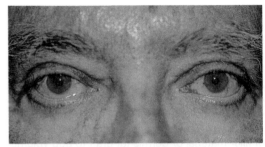

Fig. 18. Patient with postoperative lower eyelid retraction with evidence of scleral show, lateral can-thal dystopia, and periorbital hollowing. Lid retrac-tion, which develops from postsurgical manipulation, is characterized by inflammation, scar-ring, shortening, and cicatricial tethering of the middle and posterior lamella.

cicatricial ectropion, which results from exces-sive skin removal, is characterized by skin taut-ness and vertical skin tension lines. Patients with cicatricial ectropion typically present with ocular irritation from exposed, keratinized conjunctival epithelium. Lower lid ectropion worsens with mouth opening and may require a full-thickness skin graft for correction. In chronic, severe cases there may be evidence of lid retraction and cicatricial ectropion. The risks of lower lid retraction/ectropion can be decreased by using a transconjunctival approach for lower eyelid blepharoplasty, by emphasizing conservative skin removal if a trans-cutaneous infraciliary approach is performed, or using a transconjunctival/pinch technique

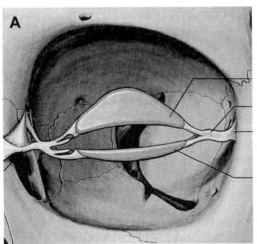
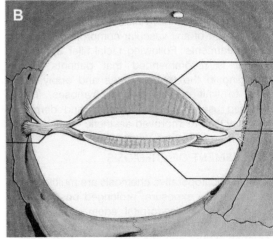

Fig. 19. (A) Eyelids: deep dissection of structural elements showing the insertion of the lateral and medial canthal tendons. (B) Eyelids: interior orbital view showing the insertion of the lateral canthal tendon as it broadens as it approaches the zygomatic rim, reaching a width of 6 to 7 mm as it inserts 1.5 mm inside the lateral bony rim. (*From* Dutton JJ. Atlas of clinical and surgical orbital anatomy. 1st edition. Philadelphia: WB Saunders; 1994; with permission.)

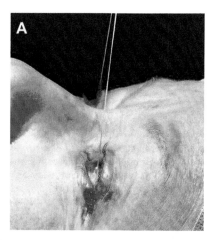

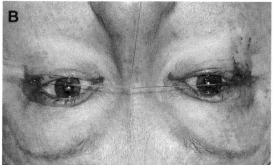

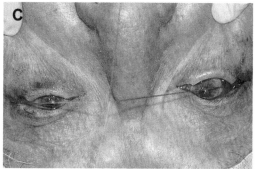

Fig. 20. Goals of lateral canthal anchoring include achieving a sharp lateral canthal angle, placement of the lid margin at the level of the limbus with no evidence of override, and vertical symmetry with the level at or slightly above the pupillary plane. (*A*) By crossing the sutures centrally before they are permanently tied, the vertical placement of the lateral canthal sutures to achieve symmetry can be verified. (*B*) Patient with evidence of asymmetrical placement of the lateral canthal anchoring sutures. (*C*) Patient with evidence of symmetric placement of the lateral canthal anchoring sutures as verified by crossing the sutures centrally. (*Courtesy of* Asa Morton, MD.)

combination. The transconjunctival incision avoids the orbital septum and therefore minimizes the risks of lower eyelid retraction from middle lamellar inflammation/scarring. The other benefit of a transconjunctival incision is that the dynamics of eyelid closure, including tear pumping and tear distribution, are not affected with preservation of the orbicularis muscle and its innervation.[12]

Conservative initial management for lower lid retraction includes massaging the area of scar contraction and the use of lubricating agents and/or steroids. It is important that even if planning reconstructive surgery following complications from prior lid surgery, the patient is treated with the medical options mentioned earlier while awaiting surgery. Lower lid laxity can be corrected by various lateral canthal anchoring procedures, including plication, canthopexy, canthoplasty, lateral retinacular

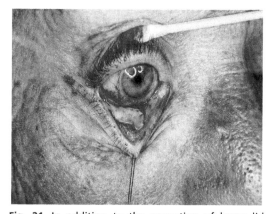

Fig. 21. In addition to the correction of lower lid laxity, the surgical repair of lower eyelid retraction requires a transconjunctival approach to completely release the scar tissue so that the eyelid is freely mobile with possible placement of a posterior lamellar spacer graft.

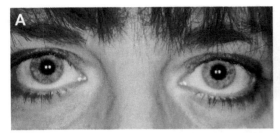
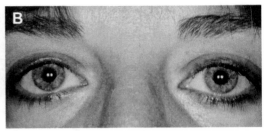

Fig. 22. (*A*) Patient with postoperative lower eyelid retraction with evidence of scleral show, lateral canthal dystopia, and periorbital hollowing. (*B*) Same patient after transconjunctival complete release of lower lid retractors with lateral canthal anchoring. It is important to reattach the lower lid inside the lateral orbital rim because the normal insertion is 1.5 mm inside the lateral orbital tubercle.

suspension, and tarsal strip procedure.[10,63–90] In lateral canthal anchoring, it is important to reattach the lower lid inside the lateral orbital rim because the normal insertion is 1.5 mm inside the lateral orbital tubercle (**Fig. 19**). If the placement is too anterior, poor apposition to the globe results, if it is too posterior, ocular irritation occurs, and if it is too superior or inferior, poor cosmesis results. The goals of lateral canthal anchoring include having sharp lateral canthal angles, positioning the lid margin at the level of the limbus with no evidence of override and by achieving vertical symmetry with the level being at or slightly above the pupillary plane. Morton has described a technique that involves crossing the sutures centrally before they are permanently tied to verify the vertical placement of the lateral canthal sutures in the correct position to achieve symmetry (**Fig. 20**).

In addition to the correction of lower lid laxity, the surgical repair of lower eyelid retraction requires a transconjunctival approach to completely release the scar tissue so that the eyelid is freely mobile with placement of a posterior lamellar spacer graft (**Figs. 21 and 22**). It is imperative to free all scarring and adhesions so that the anterior and posterior lamellar are completely mobile. This strategy allows the orbital fat to move superiorly to the normal anatomic position between the orbital septum and the capsulopalpebral fascia. Materials for posterior lamellar spacer grafts include auricular cartilage, nasal septal cartilage, porous polyethylene, sclera, tarsys, dermis fat, enduragen, and hard palate mucosal and acellular dermal grafts (see **Fig. 19**).[91–98] Acellular dermal allografts avoid the morbidity of a second operational site, as required with many of the grafts mentioned earlier; however, an increased contraction rate may be noted postoperatively. For more severe cases of lower eyelid retraction, a midface lift may be necessary in addition to the procedures described earlier.[99–103]

SUMMARY

During the initial consultation, emphasis on the importance of thorough preoperative assessment with individualized surgical planning that addresses cosmetic and functional aspects is imperative to achieve consistent aesthetic results. Before performing periocular cosmetic surgery, the surgeon should be aware of the patient's history of dry eyes, previous facial trauma, past facial surgery, previous injection of Botox Cosmetic, and history of previous LASIK. A complete evaluation should be performed on the upper eyelid/brow region for the presence of brow ptosis, eyelid ptosis, brow/eyelid asymmetry, dermatochalasis/pseudodermatochalasis, and/or deep superior sulcus. On lower eyelid/cheek examination, special attention should be directed to the diagnosis of underlying negative vector, prominent eyes, lower lid retraction, lateral canthal dystopia, scleral show, lower eyelid laxity, and lagophthalmos. In particular, emphasis on the diagnosis and treatment of underlying lower lid laxity, lid retraction, and upper lid/brow ptosis should be made by the surgeon. With upper and lower lid blepharoplasty, it is recommended that conservative skin/fat removal be emphasized, with preservation of orbicularis muscle and its innervations.

The treatment of preexisting ocular surface problems includes medical and surgical options. The medical options that can be used to treat dry eye syndrome and reduce ocular irritation include lubrication, artificial tears/ointment, topical steroids, NSAIDs, topical cyclosporine (Restasis), collage/silicone punctual plugs, and warm compresses/scrubs. These options can also be initiated in the preoperative period for patients who have planned revision surgery. If surgical correction is needed to treat postoperative complications, the following conditions may require intervention: underlying brow/eyelid ptosis, asymmetrical lid crease/fold, periorbital hollowing, deep superior sulcus, lid laxity/ectropion, and the most common functional and cosmetic problem, lower lid retraction.

Surgical rejuvenation goals in the periocular region include the avoidance of skeletonization/hollowing, repositioning and reinforcing, and avoiding deflation, with the restoration of fullness to achieve facial aesthetic balance between the forehead, eyelids, and midface. Early intervention during the postoperative period is important to correct any observed functional or cosmetic complications. With careful preoperative analysis, meticulous surgical planning and technique, the risks associated with periocular rejuvenation can be decreased or even avoided.

ACKNOWLEDGMENTS

The author wishes to thank Jennifer Barker and Barbara McGuire for their help with the manuscript.

REFERENCES

1. American Society of Plastic Surgeons (ASPS). National plastic surgery statistics. ASPS website. Available at: http://www.plasticsurgery.org/Media/stats. Accessed September 18, 2009.
2. Lyon DB, Raphits CS. Management of complications of blepharoplasty. Int Ophthalmol Clin 1997; 37(3):205–16.
3. Fulton JE. The complications of blepharoplasty: their identification and management. Dermatol Surg 1999;25(7):549–58.
4. Gausas RE. Complications of blepharoplasty. Facial Plast Surg 1999;15(3):243–53.
5. Niamtu J. Cosmetic blepharoplasty. 3rd edition. Atlas Oral Maxillofac Surg Clin North Am 2004; 12(1):91–130.
6. Morax S, Touitou V. Complications of blepharoplasty. Orbit 2006;25(4):303–18.
7. Popp JC. Complications of blepharoplasty and their management. J Dermatol Surg Oncol 1992; 18(12):1122–6.
8. Harstein ME, Kikkawa D. How to avoid blepharoplasty complications. Oral Maxillofac Surg Clin North Am 2009;21(1):31–41.
9. Knoll BI, Attkiss KJ, Persing JA. The influence of forehead, brow and periorbital aesthetics on perceived expression in the youthful face. Plast Reconstr Surg 2008;121(5):1793–802.
10. Hester TR Jr, Douglas T, Szczerba S. Decreasing complications in lower lid and midface rejuvenation: the importance of orbital morphology, horizontal lower lid laxity, history of previous surgery, and minimizing trauma to the orbital septum: a critical review of 269 consecutive cases. Plast Reconstr Surg 2009;123(3):1037–49.
11. Floegel I, Horwath-Winter J, Muellner K, et al. A conservative blepharoplasty may be a means of alleviating dry eye symptoms. Acta Ophthalmol Scand 2003;81:230.
12. Hamawy AH, Farkas JP, Fagien S, et al. Preventing and managing dry eyes after periorbital surgery: a retrospective review. Plast Reconstr Surg 2009; 123(1):353–9.
13. Vold SD, Carroll RP, Nelson JD. Dermatochalasis and dry eye. Am J Ophthalmol 1993;115:216.
14. Moss SE, Klein R, Klein BE. Prevalence of and risk factors for dry eye syndrome. Arch Ophthalmol 2000;118:1264–8.
15. Toda I, Asano-Kao N, Komai-Hori Y, et al. Dry eye after laser in situ keratomileusis. Am J Ophthalmol 2001;132:1.
16. Saadat D, Drenser SC. Safety of blepharoplasty in patients with preoperative dry eyes. Arch Facial Plast Surg 2004;6(2):101–4.
17. Fagien S. Advanced rejuvenative upper blepharoplasty: enhancing aesthetics of the upper periorbita. Plast Reconstr Surg 2002;110(1):278–91 [discussion: 292].
18. Hass AN, Penne RB, Stefanyszyn MA, et al. Incidence of post blepharoplasty orbital hemorrhage and associated visual loss. Ophthal Plast Reconstr Surg 2004;20(6):426–32.
19. Pruthi RK. Five things oculoplastic surgeons should know about the preoperative assessment of hemostasis. Ophthal Plast Reconstr Surg 2002;18(6): 396–401.
20. Teng CC, Reddy S, Wong JJ, et al. Retrobulbar hemorrhage nine days after cosmetic blepharoplasty resulting in permanent visual loss. Ophthal Plast Reconstr Surg 2006;22(5):388–9.
21. Wolfort F, Vaughan TE, Wolfort SF, et al. Retrobulbar hematoma and blepharoplasty. Plast Reconstr Surg 1999;104(7):2154–62.
22. Callahan MA. Prevention of blindness after blepharoplasty. Ophthalmology 1983;90:1047–51.
23. Goldberg RA, Marmor MF, Shorr N, et al. Blindness following blepharoplasty: two case reports and a discussion of management. Ophthalmic Surg Lasers 1990;21:81–9.
24. Mahaffey PJ, Wallace AF. Blindness following cosmetic blepharoplasty [review]. Br J Plast Surg 1986;39:213–21.
25. Putterman AM. Temporary blindness after cosmetic blepharoplasty. Am J Ophthalmol 1975;80:1081–3.
26. Jafek BW, Kreiger AE, Morledge D. Blindness following blepharoplasty. Arch Otolaryngol 1973; 98:366–9.
27. Kelly PW, May DR. Central retinal artery occlusion following cosmetic blepharoplasty. Br J Ophthalmol 1980;64:918–22.

28. Carter SR, Stewart JM, Khan J, et al. Infection after blepharoplasty with and without carbon dioxide laser resurfacing. Ophthalmology 2003; 110:1430–2.

29. Solomon KD, Fernandez deCastro LE, Sandoval P II, et al. Refractive surgery survey. J Cataract Refract Surg 2004;30:1556.

30. Shoja MR, Besharati MR. Dry eye after LASIK for myopia: incidence and risk factors. Eur J Ophthalmol 2007;17(1):1–6.

31. De Paiva CS, Cehn Z, Koch DD, et al. The incidence and risk factors for developing dry eye after myopic LASIK. Am J Ophthalmol 2006; 41(3):438–45.

32. Albietz JM, Lenton LM, McLennan SG. Dry eye after LASIK: comparison of outcomes for Asian and Caucasian eyes. Clin Exp Optom 2005;88(2):184–90.

33. Michaeli A, Slomovic AR, Sakhichand K, et al. Effect of laser in situ keratomileusis on tear secretion and corneal sensitivity. J Refract Surg 2004; 20(4):379–83.

34. Korn BS, Kikkawa DO, Schanzlin DJ. Blepharoplasty in the post-laser in situ keratomileusis patient; preoperative considerations to avoid dry eye syndrome. Plast Reconstr Surg 2007;119(7):2232–9.

35. Huang W, Rogachefsky AS, Foster JA. Brow lift with botulinum toxin. Dermatol Surg 2000;26:55–60.

36. Huilgol SC, Carruthers A, Carruthers JDA. Raising eyebrows with botulinum toxin. Dermatol Surg 2000;25:373–6.

37. Fagien S. Temporary management of upper lid ptosis, lid malposition, and eyelid fissure asymmetry with botulinum toxin. Plast Reconstr Surg 2004; 14:1892.

38. Omoigui S, Pain IS. Treatment of ptosis as a complication of botulinum toxin injection. Pain Med 2005; 6(2):149–51.

39. Wollina U, Konrad H. Managing adverse events associated with botulinum toxin type A: a focus on cosmetic procedures. Am J Clin Dermatol 2005;6(3):141–50.

40. Weinfeld AB, Burke R, Codner MA. The comprehensive management of chemosis following cosmetic lower blepharoplasty. Plast Reconstr Surg 2008;122(2):579–86.

41. Cheng JH, Lu DW. Perilimbal needle manipulation of conjunctival chemosis after cosmetic lower eyelid blepharoplasty. Ophthal Plast Reconstr Surg 2007;23(2):167–9.

42. Enzer YR, Shorr N. Medical and surgical management of chemosis after blepharoplasty. Ophthal Plast Reconstr Surg 1994;10(1):57–63.

43. Sutcliffe RT. Chemosis following blepharoplasty. Ophthalmic Surg 1995;26(4):290–1.

44. Thakker MM, Tarbet KJ, Sires BS. Postoperative chemosis after cosmetic eyelid surgery. Arch Facial Plast Surg 2005;7:185–8.

45. Syniuta LA, Goldberg RA, Thacker NM, et al. Acquired strabismus after cosmetic blepharoplasty. Plast Reconstr Surg 2003;111:2053.

46. Putterman AM. Acquired strabismus following cosmetic blepharoplasty. Plast Reconstr Surg 2004;113(3):1069–70 [author reply: 1070–1].

47. Mowlavi A, Neumeister MW, Wilhelmi BJ. Lower blepharoplasty using bony anatomical landmarks to identify and avoid injury to the inferior oblique muscle. Plast Reconstr Surg 2002;10(5):1318–22 [discussion: 1323–4].

48. Rohrich RJ, Coberly DM, Fagien S, et al. Current concepts in aesthetic upper blepharoplasty. Plast Reconstr Surg 2004;113:32e–42e.

49. Flowers RS. Blepharoplasty. In: Courtiss EH, editor. Male aesthetic surgery. St Louis (MO): CV Mosby; 1982.

50. Leone CR. Treatment of a prolapsed lacrimal gland. In: Putterman AM, editor. Cosmetic oculoplastic surgery: eyelid, forehead, and facial techniques. 3rd edition. Philadelphia: WB Saunders; 1999. p. 169–76.

51. Beer GM, Kompatscher P. A new technique for the treatment of lacrimal gland prolapse in blepharoplasty. Aesthetic Plast Surg 1994;18(1):65–9.

52. Baylis HI, Sutcliff T, Fett DR. Levator injury during blepharoplasty. Arch Ophthalmol 1984;102:570–1.

53. Burroughs JR, McLeish WM, Anderson RL. Upper blepharoplasty combined with levator aponeurosis repair. In: Fagien S, editor. Putterman's cosmetic oculoplastic surgery. 4th edition. Saunders Elsevier; 2008. p. 115–22.

54. Putterman AM, Fagien S. Muller's muscle-conjunctival resection-ptosis procedure combined with upper blepharoplasty. In: Fagien S, editor. Putterman's cosmetic oculoplastic surgery. 4th edition. Saunders Elsevier; 2008. p. 123–34.

55. Goldberg RA. Fat repositioning in lower blepharoplasty. In: Fagien S, editor. Putterman's cosmetic oculoplastic surgery. 4th edition. Saunders Elsevier; 2008. p. 217–26.

56. Trussler AP, Rohrich RJ. MOC-PS CME article: blepharoplasty. Plast Reconstr Surg 2008; 121(1):1–9.

57. Finn JC, Cox S. Fillers in the periorbital complex. Facial Plast Surg Clin North Am 2007;5(1):123–32, viii.

58. Steinsaper KD, Steinsaper SM. Deep fill hyaluronic acid for the temporary treatment of the nasojugal groove, a report on 303 consecutive treatments. Ophthal Plast Reconstr Surg 2006;5:344–8.

59. Goldberg RA, Fiaschetti B. Filling the periorbital hollows with hyaluronic gel: initial experience with the first 244 cases. Ophthal Plast Reconstr Surg 2006;22(5):335–41.

60. Fagien S, Carruthers J, Carruthers A. Injectable agents for dermal soft-tissue augmentation of the

face: options and decision making. In: Fagien S, editor. Putterman's cosmetic oculoplastic surgery. 4th edition. Saunders Elsevier; 2008. p. 279–302.

61. Putterman AM. Regarding comprehensive management of chemosis following cosmetic lower blepharoplasty. Plast Reconstr Surg 2009;124(1): 313–4.

62. Kulwin DR, Kersten RC. Blepharoplasty and brow elevation. In: Dortzbach RK, editor. Ophthalmic plastic surgery: prevention and management of complications. New York: Raven Press; 1994. p. 91–111.

63. Tenzel RR, Buffman FV, Miller G. The use of the "lateral canthal sling" ectropion repair. Can J Ophthalmol 1977;12:199.

64. Schaefer AJ. Lateral canthal tendon tuck. Am J Ophthalmol 1979;86:1879.

65. Codner MA, McCord CD, Heste TR. The lateral canthoplasty. Oper Tech Plast Reconstr Surg 1998;5:90.

66. McCord CD, Codner MA, Hester TR. Redraping the inferior orbicularis arc. Plast Reconstr Surg 1998; 102:2471.

67. Fagien S. Lower-eyelid rejuvenation via transconjunctival blepharoplasty and lateral retinacular suspension: a simplified suture canthopexy and algorithm for treatment of the anterior lower eyelid lamella. Oper Tech Plast Reconst Surg 1998;5:129.

68. Flowers RS. Canthopexy as a routine blepharoplasty component. Clin Plast Surg 1993;20:351–65.

69. Lowery JC, Bartley G. Complications of blepharoplasty. Surv Ophthalmol 1983;90:1039–46.

70. Fagien S. Algorithm for canthoplasty: the lateral retinacular suspension: a simplified suture canthopexy. Plast Reconstr Surg 1999;103:2042–53.

71. Jelks GW, Jelks EB. Repair of the lower lid deformities. Clin Plast Surg 1993;20:417.

72. Glat PM, Jelks GW, Jelks EB, et al. Evolution of the lateral canthoplasty: techniques and indications. Plast Reconstr Surg 1997;100:1396.

73. Jelks GW, Glat PM, Jelks EB, et al. The inferior retinacular lateral canthoplasty: a new technique. Plast Reconstr Surg 1997;100:1262.

74. Marsh JL, Edgerton MT. Periosteal pennant lateral canthoplasty. Plast Reconstr Surg 1979;64:24.

75. Patipa M. Lateral canthal tendon resection with conjunctiva preservation for the treatment of lower eyelid laxity during lower eyelid blepharoplasty. Plast Reconstr Surg 1993;91:456.

76. Carraway JH. The role of canthoplasty in aesthetic blepharoplasty. Aesthet Surg J 1998;18:277.

77. Rees TD. Prevention of ectropion by horizontal shortening of the lower eyelid blepharoplasty. Ann Plast Surg 1983;11:17.

78. Edgerton MT, Wolfort FG. The dermal-flap canthal lift for the lower eyelid support. Plast Reconstr Surg 1969;43:42.

79. Patipa M. The evaluation and management of lower eyelid retraction following cosmetic surgery. Plast Reconstr Surg 2000;106:438–53.

80. Millman AL, et al. The septomyocutaneous flap in lower lid blepharoplasty. Ophthal Plast Reconstr Surg 1997;13:2–6.

81. McCord CD, Shorr JW. Avoidance of complications in lower-lid blepharoplasty. Ophthalmology 1983; 90:1039–46.

82. Hinderer UT. Correction of weakness of the lower eyelid and lateral canthus. Clin Plast Surg 1993; 20:331.

83. Anderson RL, Gordy DD. The tarsal strip procedure. Arch Ophthalmol 1979;97:2192.

84. Pak J, Putterman AM. Revisional eyelid surgery: treatment of severe postblepharoplasty lower eyelid retraction. Facial Plast Surg Clin North Am 2005;13(4):461–9.

85. Lee AS, Thomas JR. Lower lid blepharoplasty and canthal surgery. Facial Plast Surg Clin North Am 2005;13(4):541–51.

86. Ativeh BS, Hayek SN. Combined arcus marginalis release, preseptal orbicularis muscle sling, and SOOF plication of midface rejuvenation. Aesthetic Plast Surg 2004;28(4):197–202.

87. Carraway JH, Grant MP, Lissauer BJ, et al. Selection of canthopexy techniques. Aesthet Surg J 2007;27(1):71–9.

88. Carraway JH, Coleman S, Kane MA, et al. Periorbital rejuvenation. Aesthet Surg J 2001;21(4): 337–43.

89. Patipa M. Transblepharoplasty lower eyelid and midface rejuvenation: part 1. Avoiding complications by utilizing lessons learned from the treatment of complications. Plast Reconstr Surg 2004;113(5): 1459–68 [discussion: 1475–7].

90. Patipa M. The evaluation and management of lower eyelid retraction following cosmetic surgery. Clin Plast Surg 2001;28:621.

91. Kersten RC, Kulwin DR, Levartovsky S, et al. Management of lower-lid retraction with hard-palate mucosa grafting. Arch Ophthalmol 1990; 108:1339–43.

92. Rubin PA, Fay AM, Remulla HD, et al. Ophthalmic plastic applications of acellular dermal allografts. Ophthalmology 1999;106:2091–7.

93. Korn BS, Kikkawa DO, Cohen SR, et al. Treatment of lower eyelid malposition with dermis fat grafting. Ophthalmology 2008;115(4):744–51.

94. Patel BC, Patipa M, Anderson RL, et al. Management of postblepharoplasty lower eyelid retraction with hard palate grafts and lateral tarsal strip. Plast Reconstr Surg 1997;99(5):1251–60.

95. Tan J, Olver J, Wright M, et al. The use of porous polyethylene (Medpor) lower eyelid spacers in lid heightening and stabilisation. Br J Ophthalmol 2004;88(9):1197–200.

96. Pang NK, Bartley GB, Bite U, et al. Hard palate mucosal grafts in oculoplastic surgery: donor site lessons. Am J Ophthalmol 2004;137(6):1021–5.

97. Oestreicher JH, Pang NK, Liao W. Treatment of lower eyelid retraction by retractor release and posterior lamellar grafting: an analysis of 659 eyelids in 400 patients. Ophthal Plast Reconstr Surg 2008;24(3):207–12.

98. McCord C, Nahai FR, Codner MA, et al. Use of porcine acellular dermal matrix (Enduragen) grafts in eyelids: a review of 69 patients and 129 eyelids. Plast Reconstr Surg 2008;122(4):1206–13.

99. Hester TR, Codner MA, McCord CD. Subperiosteal malar cheek lift with lower blepharoplasty. In: McCord CD, Codner MA, editors. Eyelid surgery. Principles and techniques. Philadelphia: Lippincott-Raven; 1995.

100. Hester TR, Codner M, McCord CD. The "centrofacial" approach for the correction of facial aging using the transblepharoplasty subperiosteal cheek lift. Aesthetic Surg Q 1996;16:51.

101. Gunter JP, Hackney FL. A simplified transblepharoplasty subperiosteal cheek lift. Plast Reconstr Surg 1999;103:2029–35.

102. Owsley JQ, Zweifler M. Midface lift of the malar fat pad: technical advances. Plast Reconstr Surg 2002;110:674.

103. Hester TR, Codner MA, McCord CD, et al. Evolution of technique of the direct transblepharoplasty approach for the correction of lower lid and midfacial aging: maximizing results and minimizing complications in a 5-year experience. Plast Reconstr Surg 2000; 105:393–406.

Index

Note: Page numbers of article titles are in **boldface** type.

facialplastic.theclinics.com

Printed and bound by CPI Group (UK) Ltd, Croydon, CR0 4YY

03/10/2024

01040356-0013